# Coming to Terms with Cancer

## Other books published by the American Cancer Society

*A Breast Cancer Journey: Your Personal Guidebook*

*American Cancer Society's Guide to Complementary and Alternative Cancer Methods*

*American Cancer Society's Guide to Pain Control*

*Cancer in the Family: Helping Children Cope with a Parent's Illness,* Heiney et al.

*Caregiving: A Step-By-Step Resource for Caring for the Person with Cancer at Home,* Houts and Bucher

*Clinical Oncology,* Lenhard et al.

*Colorectal Cancer: A Thorough and Compassionate Resource for Patients and Their Families,* Levin

*Consumers Guide to Cancer Drugs,* Wilkes et al.

*Holland-Frei Cancer Medicine,* 5th Edition, Bast et al.

*Informed Decisions,* 2nd Edition, Eyre et al.

*Our Mom Has Cancer,* Ackermann and Ackermann

*Prostate Cancer: What Every Man—and His Family—Needs to Know,* Revised Edition, Bostwick et al.

*Social Work in Oncology: Supporting Survivors, Families, and Caregivers,* Lauria et al.

*Women and Cancer: A Thorough and Compassionate Resource for Patients and Their Families,* Runowicz et al.

## Also by the American Cancer Society

*American Cancer Society's Healthy Eating Cookbook: A Celebration of Food, Friends, and Healthy Living,* 2nd Edition

*Celebrate! Healthy Entertaining for Any Occasion*

*Kids' First Cookbook: Delicious-Nutritious Treats to Make Yourself!*

# Coming to Terms with Cancer

A Glossary of Cancer-Related Terms

Edward H. Laughlin, MD

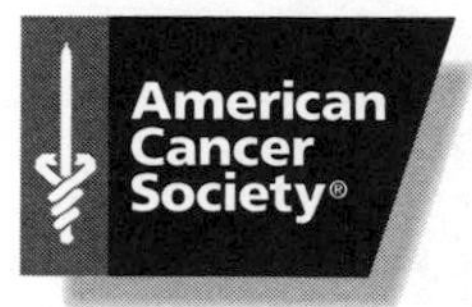

Published by
American Cancer Society
Health Content Products
1599 Clifton Road NE
Atlanta, GA 30329, USA
800-ACS-2345
http://www.cancer.org



Printed in the United States of America

5 4 3 2 1 01 02 03 04 05

**Library of Congress Cataloging-in-Publication Data**

Laughlin, Edward H.
Coming to terms with cancer : a glossary of cancer-related terminology / Edward H. Laughlin.
p. ; cm.
Includes index.
ISBN 0-944235-36-0
1. Cancer--Dictionaries.
[DNLM: 1. Neoplasms--Popular Works. 2. Neoplasms--Terminology--English. QZ 15 L374c 2001] I. Title.
RC262 .L35 2001
616.99'4'003--dc21

2001000346

**A Note to the Reader**

The information contained in this book is not intended as medical advice and should not be relied upon as a substitute for consulting with your physician. This information may not address all possible actions, precautions, side effects, or interactions. All matters regarding your health require the supervision of a physician who is familiar with your medical needs. For more information, contact your American Cancer Society at 1-800-ACS-2345 (www.cancer.org).

Book design by Mouse Design Studio, Atlanta, GA
Cover design by Jill Dible, Atlanta, GA
Illustrations (pages 1, 3, 10, 17, 35, 46, 63, 66, 110, 126, 127, 129, 136, 144, 165) by Angela Myrick

This book is dedicated in memory of James B. Laughlin, MD

and Elton Watkins, Jr., MD,

and to William H. Muller, Jr., MD.

**Managing Editor**

Katherine V. Bruss, PsyD

**Copyeditors**

Angela Myrick, BS

Jill Parsons

**Production Editor**

Thomas J. Gryczan, MS

**Editorial Review**

Herman Kattlove, MD

Len Lichtenfeld, MD

**Publishing Director**

Emily Pualwan

**Production Manager**

Candace Magee

# Contents

# Acknowledgments

I am grateful to the following physicians who reviewed specific cancers and made recommendations about treatment: Max Austin, Murray Brennan, Greg Cotter, Wyatt Fowler, Robert Ginsburg, Frank Haws, George Porter, Robert Schamberger, and Marshall Urist. This book could not have been written without the help and encouragement of Sandra Simpson, and my daughters Leedy Aboudonia, Page Easter, Hollis Volk, and Nannette Wright.

# Introduction

Cancer kills more American men and women than any other illness except heart disease. It is the second most common cause of death in children under age 15 in the United States. This year cancer will take the lives of more than 553,400 Americans of all ages. *Coming to Terms with Cancer* was written to help guide people with cancer, their families, and caregivers through the confusing maze of terminology. It is a simple to use, comprehensive glossary that includes highlights on 38 specific cancers for those who want to learn more about cancer.

The Glossary section consists of technical cancer terms, which are listed in alphabetical order and explained in language understood by most nonmedical people. The ℞ symbol indicates medications—available over-the-counter or by prescription. The Highlights section focuses on specific cancers in more detail. In this section, detailed information is offered about specific childhood and adult cancers including type of cancer and spread, risk factors, symptoms, detection, diagnosis, determining staging, and other considerations. No "preferred" treatment is given because, except for minimal or very early cancers, the treatment of malignant disease constantly changes as new treatment methods are developed. Until a "silver bullet" is devised that will treat every cancer in the same way, therapy must be individualized.

The treatment of cancer is most successful when it is detected as early as possible. It is possible to detect some cancers before symptoms occur. The American Cancer Society (ACS), along with other organizations, encourages the early detection of certain cancers before symptoms occur by recommending a cancer-related checkup and specific early detection tests for people who do not have any symptoms. The appendix lists a summary of the ACS recommendations for the early detection of cancer. A list of resources that provides contact information for a variety of organizations that offer cancer information and/or services is also included at the end of the book.

Coming to Terms with Cancer

# Glossary

## of Cancer-Related Terms

# A

**abdomen** The central part of the body, below the chest and in front of the spine, that contains the digestive organs (stomach, intestines, liver, gallbladder). The lower abdomen, surrounded by the hipbones, contains the pelvis, where the bladder, rectum, and women's reproductive organs (uterus, ovaries, fallopian tubes) lie. The abdomen is lined with peritoneum, a thin layer of tissue that also covers most abdominal organs. The space behind the abdomen is the retroperitoneum. *See also* Retroperitoneum.

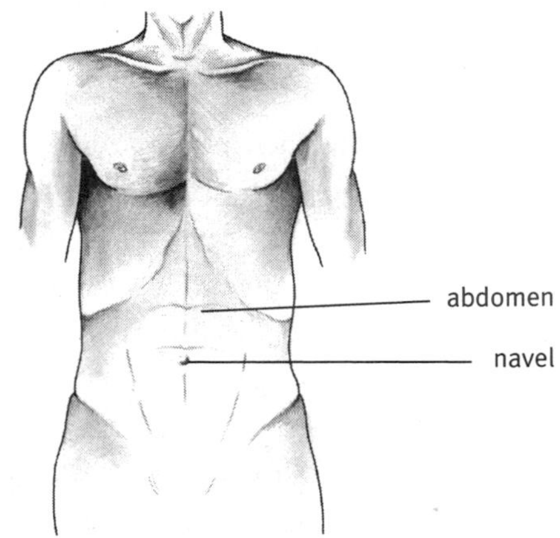


**abdominoperineal resection (APR)** The original operation for rectal and anal cancers in which the rectum, anus, and adjacent lymph nodes are removed. Because APR requires a permanent colostomy (artificial opening in the front of the abdomen) for bowel movements, newer treatments combining radiation therapy, chemotherapy, and surgery in some cases enable rectal-sparing operations, which then allow patients to have bowel movements normally, and appear to give the same treatment results. However, APR remains the standard therapy for cancer in this location. Also called Miles' resection.

**ablative therapy** A treatment that removes or destroys the function of an organ. For example, removing the ovaries or testicles or having some types of treatment that cause them to stop working.

℞ **acetaminophen** Also known by the trade name Tylenol®, this drug belongs to a group of drugs known as nonopioid analgesics (pain relievers) and antipyretics (fever reducers).

℞ **Achromycin®** *See* Tetracycline Hydrochloride.

**acoustic neuroma** A benign (noncancerous) brain tumor of the major nerve to the ear (acoustic or cranial nerve VIII). The usual operation to completely remove the tumor may cause deafness, weakness of the face, and/or difficulty with balance. Newer treatment methods that combine radiation with surgery that only partially removes the tumor give the same results as surgery that completely removes the growth. Also called acoustic schwannoma; cerebellopontine angle tumor; acoustic neurilemoma.

**acoustic schwannoma** *See* Acoustic Neuroma.

**acquired immunodeficiency syndrome (AIDS)** A group of fatal medical disorders caused by human immunodeficiency virus-1 (HIV-1), which destroys the body's immune (protective) mechanism. HIV is spread through blood and body fluids, and can be passed from an infected mother to her unborn child. People infected with HIV are considered to have AIDS if they acquire an unusual infection, such as *Pneumocystis carinii* pneumonia, fungal infections with candida, or develop a particular cancer such as Kaposi's sarcoma or lymphoma of the brain.

The first malignancy recognized as part of AIDS was Kaposi's sarcoma, previously a rare skin cancer most often found on the legs in elderly Jewish men and men of Mediterranean descent. Although about 95% of males who develop this cancer today are either homosexual or bisexual men with AIDS, Kaposi's sarcoma has become less common in gay men compared to the 1980s when AIDS was first recognized. Unlike Kaposi's sarcoma that most often affects men, brain lymphoma occurs equally in both sexes, although female intravenous (IV) drug abusers who are HIV-positive are less likely to develop lymphoma than are their male counterparts. Unfortunately, brain lymphoma often occurs in AIDS patients who initially respond to treatment, and appear to be doing well. Since 1993, HIV-positive women who develop cervical cancer are considered to have AIDS.

Most cancers associated with HIV infections tend to grow faster and involve internal organs more often than do similar malignancies in non-HIV infected people. This probably occurs as a result of the body's compromised immune system rather than a direct effect of the virus. *See also* Kaposi's Sarcoma; Non-Hodgkin's Lymphoma (pages 188–190).

**acral lentiginous** *See* Melanoma (pages 182–184).

℞ **acridinyl anisidide** *See* Amsacrine and AMSA P-D®.

**ACTH** Adrenocorticotropic hormone is produced by the pituitary gland at the base of the brain. It stimulates the outer part (cortex) of both adrenal glands to release different hormones, such as cortisol (a steroid hormone), which regulates body metabolism and levels of glucose (sugar) and minerals (sodium and potassium) in the blood. Both lung and pancreatic cancers can sometimes produce ACTH and cause the adrenal glands to release excess hydrocortisone. This results in Cushing's syndrome, a medical condition that is characterized by a round face, obesity of the trunk, stretch marks on the abdominal skin, a tendency to diabetes, and high blood pressure or hypertension. *See also* Pituitary.

℞ **Actinomycin D®** *See* Dactinomycin.

℞ **Actiq®** *See* Fentanyl Citrate.

**acute** Any disease or medical disorder of sudden onset, which usually denotes a severe problem (acute leukemia, acute appendicitis). The opposite of chronic or long-standing.

℞ **acyclovir** Also known by the trade name Zovirax®, this drug belongs to a group of drugs known as antiviral agents. It is used to treat infections with herpes simplex virus, herpes zoster virus, and cytomegalovirus.

**adenocarcinoma** A cancer that forms in glands or gland-like tissue; the usual variety of malignant tumor found in the breast, colon, rectum, and ovary. It is also a common primary cancer in the lung.

**adenoma** A usually well-defined, benign (noncancerous) tumor of epithelial tissue that starts in the glandular tissue. Among the more common adenomas are fibroadenoma of the breast and follicular adenoma of the thyroid gland.

**adjuvant therapy** Cancer treatment using chemotherapy, hormone therapy, or radiation therapy after a cancer operation (or other treatment) to enhance the effects of the initial treatment. *See also* Neoadjuvant Therapy.

**adrenal cortical insufficiency** Failure of the adrenal gland cortex to produce cortisol (and other hormones). Acute adrenal insufficiency will occur rapidly following total surgical adrenalectomy. It can also occur in patients who have been treated with oral prednisone and similar medications, and becomes a problem after those medicines are discontinued. Some medications used rarely in the treatment of cancer can cause the adrenal gland to stop functioning altogether, which is termed a "medical adrenalectomy." Adrenal cortical insufficiency is fatal unless it is recognized and treated with hydrocortisone.

**adrenal gland** One of a pair of small glands that are attached to the top of each kidney, which produce a variety of essential hormones. Each is composed of two distinct parts: an inner portion (medulla) that produces the hormone epinephrine, which among other actions increases heart rate and blood pressure; and an outer layer (cortex) that produces small amounts of the weak, male sex hormone, androstenedione, and cortisol, a hormone that controls levels of glucose (sugar) and minerals (sodium, potassium) in the blood. These glands rarely give rise to both cancerous and noncancerous tumors. Non-small cell lung cancer (NSCLC) frequently spreads to the adrenal glands.

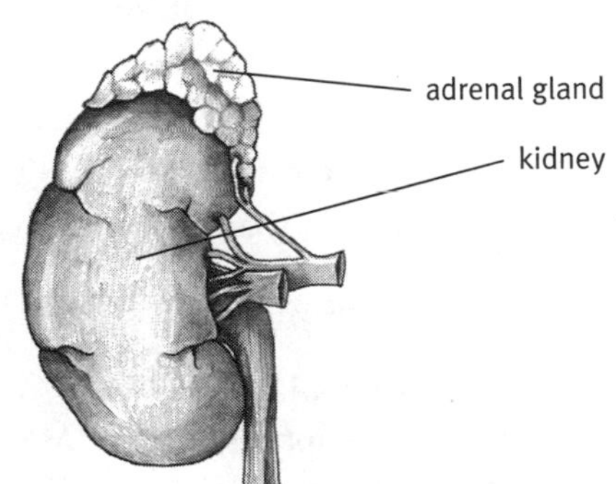

**adrenalectomy** Surgical removal of one or both adrenal glands. Removal of one adrenal gland (unilateral) is used to treat a tumor that has started in the gland or, less often, has spread there from a cancer elsewhere in the body.

**adrenaline** This is the potent hormone epinephrine, produced in the inner portion (medulla) of both adrenal glands, whose actions include increased pulse (heart rate) and blood pressure. Epinephrine when mixed with local anesthetic drugs, such as lidocaine, prolongs anesthesia. *See* Epinephrine.

℞ **Adriamycin®** *See* Doxorubicin.

**advance directives** Legal documents that tell the physician and family what a person wants for future medical care, including whether to start or when to stop life-sustaining treatment.

**advanced cancer** A general term describing the stages of cancer in which the disease has spread from the primary site to other parts of the body. When the cancer has spread only to the surrounding areas, it is called locally advanced. If it has spread further by traveling through the bloodstream or lymph system, it is called metastatic.

℞ **Advil®** *See* Ibuprofen.

**aflatoxin** A carcinogen (cancer-causing substance) from fungi (*Aspergillus*) contaminating grain and peanuts raised in warm, wet climates, and stored in hot, damp surroundings. Aflatoxin, together with viral hepatitis, appears responsible for the large numbers of cases of liver cancer (hepatocellular carcinoma or liver cell cancer) found in Equatorial Africa.

**afterbirth** *See* Placenta.

**afterloading** A type of treatment used in cancer radiation therapy (called brachytherapy) in which the radiation source is placed in tubes or in a device previously positioned in or near a tumor. After the calculated radiation dose is given, the tubes and radioactive sources are usually removed. However, in some types of treatment, such as for prostate cancer, the radioactive seeds may be left permanently in place. The technique is used to treat a variety of malignant tumors that include breast, prostate, and head and neck cancers.

**agent** Any substance or force able to affect the body.

℞ **AG3340** Also known by the trade name Prinomastat®, this drug is a matrix metalloproteinase (MMP) inhibitor. MMPs are enzymes that help tumor cells to grow, invade surrounding tissue, and develop blood vessels that help cancer cells to spread to distant tissues. This drug prevents the action of these enzymes so that tumor cells do not grow or spread to other tissues. This falls within a new class of drugs called "antiangiogenesis drugs" and several are in the early stages of development and/or clinical trials. *See* Angiogenesis.

**AIDS** *See* Acquired Immunodeficiency Syndrome.

℞ **alemtuzumab** Also known by the trade name Campath®, this drug is a monoclonal antibody used for the treatment of patients with B cell chronic lymphocytic leukemia (B-CLL) whose cancer is not responding to first line chemotherapy. Its target on the leukemia cell is a protein known as CD52, which is present on leukemic B lymphocytes.

**alimentary canal** *See* Digestive Tract.

℞ **alitretinoin gel 0.1%** Also known by the trade name Panretin®, this drug binds to certain retinoid receptors on cancer cells to control their growth and division. (Receptors are microscopic places on the surfaces of cells that respond to certain signals from other substances in the body.) The medication has been found to stop the growth of Kaposi's sarcoma (KS) cells, and is used for the treatment of KS skin lesions. *See also* Kaposi's Sarcoma.

**alkaline phosphatase** An enzyme in blood that is increased in both cancer and noncancerous diseases of bone and liver. Elevated levels in cancer patients are frequently signs of spread of a cancer to the bone and/or liver.

**alkylating agent** Any one of a variety of chemotherapy drugs that includes mechlorethamine (nitrogen mustard—the first drug, other than hormones, used to treat cancer effectively and consistently), melphalan, chlorambucil, cyclophosphamide, and nitrosoureas. They are used for a variety of malignancies, including lymphoma, leukemia, and brain tumors. All are toxic to bone marrow, and may cause anemia, infection, or bleeding. Some of these drugs are given intravenously, others by mouth, and some by either route.

**allogenic, allogeneic** The term to describe a tissue graft or an organ transplant in which the donor, usually a relative, is genetically similar, but not identical to the recipient.

℞ **allopurinol** Also known by the trade names Zyloprim®, Alprim®, and Zurinol®, this drug blocks xanthine oxidase, the enzyme necessary for making uric acid. When cancer cells are killed, they release substances that increase the production of uric acid (tumor lysis syndrome), which can damage the kidneys. This drug is used in the initial treatment of patients with leukemia, lymphoma, and small cell lung cancer. It is also commonly used in the treatment of patients with gout and/or elevated levels of uric acid.

**alopecia** Loss of hair, especially of the scalp. This is a common, distressing side effect of both chemotherapy (especially the drug doxorubicin), and radiation therapy to the head. Hair loss due to chemotherapy is almost always reversible after treatment is stopped, although the color and texture of the new growth may be different. However, alopecia from radiation to the head is unpredictable, and may be permanent. *Look Good...Feel Better,* a program of the American Cancer Society, has volunteers who can help people with cancer cope with hair loss during treatment (*see* Resources section following Appendix).

Rx **Aloprim®** *See* Allopurinol.

**alpha blocker** A drug that relaxes smooth muscle tissue. It is commonly used in the treatment of hypertension and relief of prostate obstruction symptoms in men. *See also* Benign Prostatic Hypertrophy.

**alpha-fetoprotein** A type of protein produced by the fetus that is present in small amounts in the blood of adults. Used as a tumor marker in liver cancer (hepatocellular cancer in adults, hepatoblastoma in children) and yolk sac tumor, which is a type of cancer that may start in the ovaries and testicles.

**alpha ray** A form of solar radiation that together with beta rays make up ultraviolet (UV) radiation from the sun; both of which appear to cause skin cancer (melanoma). Only sunscreens that block both alpha and beta rays adequately protect from sun exposure, and the recommended minimal sun protection factor (SPF) is 15.

Rx **alprazolam** Also known by the trade name Xanax®, this is an anxiolytic (anxiety reliever) that belongs to a group of drugs known as benzodiazepines. It is also used in the treatment of panic attacks.

**alternative therapy** Use of an unproven therapy instead of standard (proven) therapy. Some alternative therapies have dangerous or even life-threatening side effects. For others, the main danger is that a patient may lose the opportunity to benefit from standard therapy. *See also* Unproven Treatment.

Rx **altretamine** Also known by the trade names Hexalen® and Hexamethylmelamine®, this drug belongs to a group of drugs known as alkylating agents. It is used to treat several types of cancer, including ovarian cancer.

**alveoli** The small air sacs in the lung where oxygen is exchanged for carbon dioxide. In emphysema, a disease caused by smoking, the thin walls of the alveoli collapse and cause large pockets to form, making it more difficult to take oxygen into the body and in turn causing shortness of breath. *See also* Lung Cancer (pages 180–182).

℞ **Ambien®** *See* Zolpidem Tartrate.

℞ **Amdray®** *See* Valspodar.

℞ **Amethopterin®** *See* Methotrexate.

℞ **amifostine** Also known by the trade name Ethyol®, this is an intravenous drug used to reduce injury to the kidneys from repeated administration of cisplatin in patients with advanced ovarian cancer or non-small cell lung cancer. The most severe adverse effect is hypotension (low blood pressure) in people who are dehydrated or who are taking medication for high blood pressure.

℞ **amikacin sulfate** Also known by the trade name Amikin®, this is an antibiotic that belongs to a group of drugs known as aminoglycosides. Its major side effect is kidney damage, so drug levels in the blood must be monitored carefully.

℞ **Amikin®** *See* Amikacin Sulfate.

℞ **9-aminocamptothecin (9-AC)** This investigational drug belongs to a group of drugs known as topisomerase inhibitors. It has been studied in the treatment of several types of cancer, including colon and ovarian cancers.

℞ **aminoglutethimide** Also known by the trade names Cytadren® and Elipten®, this drug is used infrequently as hormone therapy in advanced breast cancer. It blocks production of several hormones, including cortisol, estrogen, and androgen from the outer part (cortex) of the adrenal glands. It also prevents the conversion of estrogen from androstenedione, a weak male hormone secreted by the adrenal glands. This chemical conversion occurs in subcutaneous tissue (fatty tissue under the skin), and is the source of estrogen in postmenopausal women.

℞ **aminoglycosides** A group of antibiotics used to treat severe bacterial infections. They inhibit the growth of bacteria.

℞ **amitriptyline hydrochloride** Also known by the trade name Elavil®, this drug belongs to a group of drugs known as tricyclic antidepressants. In addition to relieving depression, it is used to help patients with chronic pain.

℞ **amoxicillin** Also known by the trade name Amoxil®, this drug is an antibiotic used to treat bacterial infections of the respiratory, genital, and urinary tracts. It is part of the penicillin family.

℞ **amoxicillin combined with clavulanate** Also known by the trade name Augmentin®, this drug is a penicillin-related antibiotic used to treat bacterial infections of the respiratory, genital, and urinary tract that do not respond to penicillin alone.

℞ **Amoxil®** *See* Amoxicillin.

℞ **amphotericin B (amphotericin B lipid complex)** Also known by the trade name Fungizone®, this is an antifungal and antiprotozoal agent. It is used to treat fungal infections in the blood and spinal cord.

℞ **ampicillin sodium combined with sulbactam** Also known by the trade name Unasyn®, this antibiotic drug is used to treat bacterial infections of the respiratory, genital, and urinary tracts.

**ampulla of vater** The lower end of the tube-like common bile duct through which bile drains from the liver into the duodenum, the upper part of the small intestine. Because cancer of the ampulla blocks the flow of bile and causes jaundice, it is often confused by physicians with the more common and deadly pancreatic cancer. Treatment for ampullary cancer is the Whipple operation or radical pancreatoduodenectomy. *See also* Head of Pancreas; Whipple Operation.

**amputate** To surgically remove all or part of a limb (arm, leg) or a raised body part (breast, nose).

℞ **AMSA P-D®** *See* Amsacrine.

℞ **amsacrine** Also known as acridinyl anisidide and by the trade name AMSA P-D®, this drug belongs to a group of drugs known as topisomerase inhibitors. It is used to treat several types of cancer, including leukemia and lymphoma.

**anal** Relating to the anus. *See* Anal Cancer (pages 152–153).

**analog** A synthetic version of a naturally-occurring substance.

**anaplastic cancer** Any rapidly growing cancer where the cells (when examined under a microscope) do not resemble normal cells of the organ or site in which the malignancy arises. Also called undifferentiated cancer.

**anastomosis** The site where two structures are surgically joined together, such as the bladder neck and the urethra after removal of the prostate.

℞ **anastrozole** Also known by the trade name Arimidex®, this drug is used as hormone therapy for recurrent breast cancer that is estrogen receptor-positive (ER+) in postmenopausal women previously treated with tamoxifen (Nolvadex®). It also prevents androstenedione, the weak male hormone produced in the adrenal glands of both sexes, from being converted into the female hormone in fatty tissue (subcutaneous tissue) under the skin.

℞ **Ancel®** *See* Cefazolin Sodium.

℞ **Ancobon®** *See* Flucytosine.

**androgen** Any hormone or other substance that produces masculine traits, including development of sex organs, body build, hair pattern, and depth of voice. The most potent androgen, testosterone, is produced in the testicle (testes). The less active hormone, androstenedione, is produced not only in the testes but also in the adrenal cortex and ovaries. Removing the main source of androgen, either by castration or giving medication such as goserelin, is used in treating advanced-stage prostate cancer.

**androgen ablation** *See* Combination Hormone Therapy.

**androgen blockade** *See* Combination Hormone Therapy.

**androgen dependent** Prostate cells, benign or malignant, that are stimulated to grow and multiply by male hormones and are suppressed by drugs that disrupt the action of male hormones.

**anemia** A condition resulting either from decreased numbers of red blood cells (RBCs) or reduced iron content in RBCs. Symptoms depend on the degree of anemia and vary from paleness and fatigue in mild cases to shortness of breath, weakness, and irregular heart beat in extreme situations. Anemia due to bleeding in the digestive tract may be the first indication of colon cancer. Malignant disease affecting bone marrow, including leukemia, many types of chemotherapy, and poor nutrition all affect RBCs by affecting the growth of cells in the bone marrow where red blood cells are produced. Pernicious anemia is caused by the stomach's failure to absorb vitamin $B_{12}$. It can also occur after gastrectomy (complete removal of the stomach). Vegetarians need to be certain they have enough $B_{12}$ in their diet to avoid developing pernicious anemia.

℞ **Anergan®** *See* Promethazine Hydrochloride.

**anesthesia** The loss of feeling or sensation as a result of drugs or gases. General anesthesia causes loss of consciousness. Local, regional, or spinal anesthesia numbs only a specific area.

**angiogenesis** The development of new blood vessels that enables cancers to grow and that allows malignant cells to be carried through blood to distant sites or organs, where they can develop into secondary cancer(s) or metastasis. *See also* Antiangiogenesis.

**aniline dye** Any one of a number of synthetic dyes usually made from coal tar; known to cause bladder cancer in exposed workers. *See also* Carcinogen.

**anorexia** The loss of appetite that may be caused by either the cancer itself or as a side effect of treatment such as chemotherapy.

℞ **Anspor®** *See* Cephradine.

**antiangiogenesis** Experimental cancer treatment that prevents the development of blood vessels (angiogenesis) in malignant tumors. Because angiogenesis is necessary for tumor growth, antiangiogenesis drugs, if successful, should prevent the growth of micrometastases (very small tumors) from advanced cancers and should shrink large tumors. Several antiangiogenesis drugs are now in clinical trials for cancer patients. *See also* Angiogenesis.

℞ **antibiotic** A substance from molds and bacteria that stops the growth of other bacteria (antibacterial), fungi (antifungal), or cancer cells (antitumor). One of the antibiotics most often used in cancer chemotherapy is doxorubicin. Since some cancer treatments can reduce the body's ability to fight off infection, antibiotics may be used to treat or prevent these infections. You should discuss the use of antibiotics with your physician if you have an allergy to penicillin.

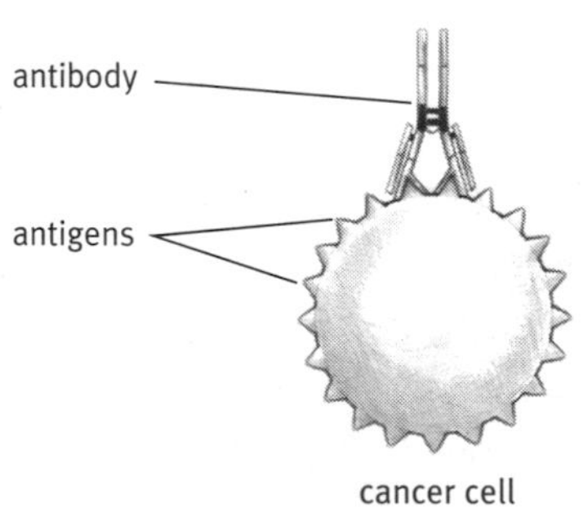


**antibody** A specialized protein molecule in the blood; part of the body's immune system that protects against infection. A distinct antibody is produced in response to contact with a specific chemical molecule (antigen) introduced or formed in the body. Antibodies can also be used in the laboratory, where they can identify cancer cells or markers in tissue examined under the microscope. They are also being used as cancer treatments, *see* Rituximab; Trastuzumab.

℞ **anticoagulant** This refers to an agent that delays coagulation (blood clotting). It is used both to prevent and treat blood clots that often occur in cancer patients. The two most widely used anticoagulants are heparin, given by injection, and warfarin, given by mouth or injection. All can cause severe bleeding, and their effects need to be monitored closely using the clotting time or activated prothrombin test (APTT) for heparin, and the prothrombin time (PT) for warfarin. Many drugs (including aspirin) taken with these agents can cause serious problems, including increasing the risk of bleeding (such as aspirin or other nonsteroidal drugs) or increasing their anticlotting effect. It is very important to monitor the effects of these drugs and to follow your health care provider's instructions when taking these medications. *See also* Heparin; Warfarin.

℞ **antiemetic** A drug that prevents or relieves nausea or vomiting, which are common side effects of chemotherapy.

℞ **antiestrogen** A substance that blocks the effects of estrogen on tumors, such as the drug tamoxifen. Antiestrogens work best when they are used to treat breast cancer that depends on estrogen for growth.

**antigen** Any substance that causes the formation of a specific antibody after exposure to it. Specific antigens on the surface of red blood cells identify blood type, and antigens on cancer cells can help to accurately identify cancer types.

℞ **anti-HER2/*neu*** *See* Trastuzumab.

℞ **antimetabolite** Any one of several drugs, including methotrexate and fluorouracil (5-FU), widely used in cancer chemotherapy. All affect rapidly growing cancer cells by interfering with the chemical substances (metabolites) necessary for cell growth and reproduction. *See* Fluorouracil; Methotrexate.

**antioxidants** Molecules, such as some vitamins, that block the actions of activated oxygen molecules, known as free radicals that can damage cells.

**anus** The body opening at the lower end of the intestinal tract through which solid waste is passed.

℞ **Anzemet®** *See* Dolasetron Mesylate.

℞ **Apo-Prednisone®** *See* Prednisone.

**apoptosis** The orderly mechanism, referred to by physicians as "programmed cell death," by which normal cells die after a finite period. Apoptosis is reduced in cancer cells, which stop growing only with effective treatment or with the death of the individual harboring the cancer. Apoptosis can be brought about by some drugs used to treat cancer.

**APTT** Activated partial thromboplastin time is a laboratory test that measures the time it takes blood plasma to form a clot following the addition of calcium and another reagent (phospholipid). It is used to evaluate and monitor blood clotting and anticoagulant therapy.

℞ **Aredia®** *See* Pamidronate Disodium.

**areola** The dark area of skin that surrounds the nipple of the breast.

℞ **Arimidex®** *See* Anastrozole.

℞ **Aromasin®** *See* Exemestane.

**artificial sphincter** An inflatable cuff implanted around the upper urethra to squeeze the urethra shut and provide urinary control.

**asbestos** A mineral fiber particularly associated with lung cancer and with pleural mesothelioma, a cancer of the lining of the chest. Once widely used for insulating houses and buildings and lining brake shoes, it is no longer used because it is hazardous to workers exposed over many years, especially to those who smoke. *See also* Carcinogen; Lung Cancer (pages 180–182); Mesothelioma (pages 184–185).

**ascending colon** The first of four sections of the colon. It extends upward on the right side of the abdomen. *See also* Colon.

**ascites** Accumulation of fluid in the abdomen, which can cause painful abdominal swelling and difficult breathing; often caused by intra-abdominal malignancies, especially ovarian cancer. It also occurs in patients with advanced cirrhosis of the liver. Accumulation of ascitic fluid not controlled by a diuretic drug can be removed either by paracentesis (needle puncture) or an internal shunt (Denver® shunt, LeVeen shunt) that diverts abdominal fluid into a vein, where blood carries it to the kidneys for removal in urine. *See also* Denver® Shunt; LeVeen Shunt; Paracentesis.

℞ **asparaginase** Also known by the trade name Elspar®, this drug is an enzyme used to treat several types of cancer, including acute leukemia.

℞ **aspirin (acetylsalicylic acid)** This is a nonopioid analgesic that belongs to a group of drugs known as salicylates. It is also known as a nonsteroidal anti-inflammatory drug (NSAID). This drug blocks the synthesis of prostaglandins, preventing pain receptors from passing pain messages to the brain. It also prevents inflammation and reduces fever. It has also been shown to possibly reduce the risk of developing certain cancers, such as colon cancer.

**Astler-Coller staging system** One of the staging systems for colon and rectal cancer. In this system, the letters A through D are used for the various stages, with "A" representing an early-stage lesion and "D" representing advanced, metastatic disease.

℞ **Astramorph®** *See* Morphine.

**astrocytoma** A common brain tumor that affects both children and adults. It can vary from a very slow growing, essentially benign variety, to a rapidly expanding growth called a glioblastoma multiforme that is usually fatal in less than 2 years. *See* Brain Tumor (pages 157–159).

**asymptomatic** Not having any symptoms of a disease. Many cancers develop and grow without producing symptoms, especially in the early stages.

℞ **Ativan®** *See* Lorazepam.

℞ **Atragen®** *See* Liposomal Tretinoin.

**atypical** A term meaning not usual; abnormal. Often refers to the appearance of cancerous or precancerous cells.

**atypical hyperplasia** A term used most often to describe thickening of the cell layers in the breast in either the very small lobular ducts (atypical lobular hyperplasia) or large milk ducts (atypical ductal hyperplasia). Although it is benign (noncancerous), women with atypical hyperplasia, especially those with a family history of breast cancer, have a moderately increased risk of later developing breast cancer.

℞ **Augmentin®** *See* Amoxicillin Combined with Clavulanate.

**autologous** The term to describe a tissue transplant in which the donor and recipient are the same individual. This includes skin graft, bone marrow or stem cell graft, and blood transfusion.

℞ **Aventyl®** *See* Nortriptyline Hydrochloride.

℞ **5AZ®** *See* 5-azacytidine.

℞ **Azactam®** *See* Aztreonam.

℞ **5-azacytidine** Also known by the trade names Azacytidine® and 5AZ®, this drug belongs to a group of drugs known as antimetabolites. It is used to treat several types of cancer, including acute myelocytic leukemia.

℞ **Azacytidine®** *See* 5-azacytidine.

℞ **azithromycin** Also known by the trade name Zithromax®, this is an antibiotic used to treat bacterial infections. It is related to the erythromycin class of drugs, and the usual course of treatment is shorter than with many other antibiotics.

℞ **aztreonam** Also known by the trade name Azactam®, this drug is an antibiotic.

# B

℞ **Bactocill®** *See* Oxacillin Sodium.

℞ **Bactrim®** *See* Co-Trimoxazole (Trimethoprim and Sulfamethoxazole).

**baldness** *See* Alopecia.

**barium enema** An x-ray examination of the large intestine (colon, rectum) to diagnose cancer, polyps (noncancerous growths), and diseases such as chronic ulcerative colitis and diverticulosis. An enema containing air and barium sulfate, a compound opaque to x-rays, is gently pumped into the rectum during which x-ray pictures are taken of the abdomen. To ensure an accurate reading, a clear liquid diet (Jell-O®, broth, tea, coffee) is taken for 24 hours before the study, and a laxative is given the night before. Also called double contrast barium enema.

**barium swallow** An x-ray examination of the esophagus (swallowing tube located in the chest) to detect diseases or problems, including strictures and esophageal cancer, among others. A liquid containing barium sulfate, a compound opaque to x-rays, is swallowed during which x-ray pictures are taken of the chest.

**Barrett's esophagus** A premalignant condition associated with adenocarcinoma of the lower end of the esophagus in which the esophagus is lined with columnar epithelium that resembles the mucosa (lining) of the gastric cardia (upper portion of the stomach). It is caused by esophagitis (persistent irritation) due to refluxing (stomach acid flowing) up into the esophagus. Persistent reflux symptoms (heartburn, acid taste) should prompt esophagoscopy and biopsy to detect this condition, which, if present, requires regular and repeated esophagoscopy to detect early cancer. *See also* Esophageal Cancer (pages 167–168).

**basal cell carcinoma** A slow growing and frequent skin cancer of older people, which occurs most often on sun-exposed areas (face, neck, ears, scalp, arms), usually as a slightly raised growth with a depressed center. It very seldom spreads to lymph nodes, but left untreated, basal cell cancer can enlarge, and in some cases, grow into and destroy surrounding tissue, including bone. Small cancers are easily cured by surgery, fluorouracil (5-FU), chemotherapy cream (Efudex®), cryotherapy (freezing), or cautery (electric current). *See also* Skin Cancer (pages 199–201).

**B cell** A type of white blood cell (lymphocyte); part of the body's immune (protective) mechanism that produces different antibodies. B cells develop in lymph-containing tissues from stem cells that have migrated from their origin in bone marrow. They can develop into lymphoma and leukemia. *See also* Lymphocyte.

**BCG** Bacillus Calmette-Guérin is a vaccine made from the bacteria *Mycobacterium bovis,* the primary cause of tuberculosis in cattle, which was developed to prevent tuberculosis in humans. It is effective in treating human cancer by stimulating the body's immune system (natural defenses). BCG is currently used as immunotherapy for melanoma that recurs in skin as well as in early-stage bladder cancer.

Rx **BCNU®** *See* Nitrosourea.

Rx **Benadryl®** *See* Diphenhydramine Hydrochloride.

**benign** A term that signifies any mild type of illness or medical condition. It is most often used to describe a nonmalignant (noncancerous) tumor.

**benign prostatic hypertrophy or hyperplasia (BPH)** A noncancerous enlargement of the prostate gland that normally affects older men. BPH can cause urinary problems (frequent urination, difficulty starting urination, weak urinary stream) similar to those caused by prostate cancer. Any man experiencing any of these symptoms should be evaluated by a urologist or other knowledgeable physician. It can be treated with oral medications and/or surgery.

**beta carotene** A nutritional substance in carrots and yellow vegetables that is converted by the body into vitamin A. It is thought to protect against certain cancers. A recent study involving thousands of physicians who took beta carotene regularly for 10 years found no evidence that it protects against colon cancer. However, the compound is being investigated as a preventive for other cancers (lung, stomach, esophagus).

**beta human chorionic gonadotropin (β-hCG)** A hormone produced by the placenta (membranes of pregnancy; afterbirth) as well as by some malignant tumors. It is used as a tumor marker to indicate the presence of certain cancers (choriocarcinoma and some mixed germ cell tumors) of the testis, ovary, and placenta.

**beta ray** A type of ultraviolet ray from the sun (solar radiation) that causes tanning and sunburn. It has been implicated in the development of melanoma and skin cancer. Only sunscreens with a sun protection factor (SPF) of at least 15 that protects from both beta rays and weaker alpha rays provide adequate protection from the sun.

Rx **bexarotene** Also known by the trade name Targretin®, this drug activates certain retinoid receptors. A retinoid is a naturally-occurring substance that regulates or controls certain genes to help cells grow and divide. Bexarotene activates certain retinoid receptors on the cell, and these receptors work with other substances to control the growth and division of cancer cells. It is used in the treatment of skin lesions due to cutaneous T cell lymphoma that have not responded to prior systemic treatment.

Rx **Bexxar®** *See* Tositumomab.

Rx **bicalutamide** Also known by the trade name Casodex®, this drug is a hormone antagonist (a nonsteroidal antiandrogen). It is used in the treatment of advanced prostate cancer, and blocks the effects of testosterone on prostate cancer cells.

Rx **BiCNU®** *See* Nitrosourea.

**bilateral** On both sides of the body; for example, bilateral breast cancer is cancer in both breasts at the same time (synchronous) or at different times (metachronous).

**bile** A clear, green-yellow fluid from the liver that flows through the tube-like common bile duct into the duodenum (upper small intestine) where it mixes with food and aids in digesting fats. Jaundice (yellow staining of skin and eyes) due to obstruction of bile flow is often the first symptom of cancers of the pancreas, liver, biliary duct, and gallbladder. *See also* Bile Duct Cancer (pages 153–154).

**biliary** Relating either to bile or to the system that conveys bile (bile ducts in the liver, common bile duct, and gallbladder).

**biologic response modifiers** Substances that boost the body's immune system to fight against cancer.

**biologic therapy** *See* Immunotherapy.

**biomarkers** *See* Tumor Markers.

**biopsy** The process of removing a tissue or fluid sample for examination under the microscope; used to diagnose cancer and other diseases. Also, the sample (specimen) itself (lung biopsy, skin biopsy). There are several biopsy techniques:

*Pap test:* This simple procedure obtains cells scraped from the body (most often cervix) from fluid present in a cyst, or from a body cavity such as the abdomen or chest.

*Needle biopsy:* Tissue samples are obtained using a needle inserted into a mass or lump. Fine needle aspiration (FNA) provides a fluid or tissue sample drawn up through a very small needle, whereas core needle (Trucut needle) provides a ¾-inch long tissue sample about the diameter of a toothpick. If a mass cannot be felt or lies deep within the body, the needle is positioned using CT or ultrasound. The advantages of FNA are that it is relatively painless, safe, inexpensive, and does not spread tumor cells. However, the tissue sample obtained is small and may not be sufficient for diagnosis. Core needle (Trucut) biopsy is generally used to sample prostate, liver, and large tumors. It is important to remember that any biopsy reported as "negative for cancer" means only that malignant cells are not seen in the specimen analyzed, so cancer may still be present elsewhere in the body.

*Incisional biopsy:* This surgically removes a portion of mass or tumor, and is often used during operations to both diagnose and stage cancer.

*Excisional biopsy:* A procedure to remove an entire growth; often the only treatment necessary for small tumors.

*See also* Core Needle Biopsy; Excisional Biopsy; Fine Needle Aspiration; Incisional Biopsy; Stereotactic Breast Biopsy.

℞ **bisacodyl** Also known by the trade name Dulcolax®, this drug belongs to a group of drugs known as stimulant laxatives. It is used to relieve constipation.

℞ **Blenoxane®** *See* Bleomycin Sulfate.

℞ **bleomycin sulfate** Also known by the trade name Blenoxane®, this antibiotic type of chemotherapy drug is used for a variety of malignancies including head and neck cancer, lymphoma, and testicular cancer. It is also used to treat pleural effusion (recurring fluid in the chest) by injecting it into the space between the lung and inside of the chest wall. The most serious side effect of intravenous (IV) bleomycin is a scarring of the lung tissue called pulmonary fibrosis. It is usually related to the cumulative dose of bleomycin received by the patient.

**blood-brain barrier** A selective mechanism of capillaries (small blood vessels) in the brain that inhibits chemical compounds, including most chemotherapy drugs, from passing from blood into brain tissue.

**blood count** A count of the number of red blood cells, white blood cells, and platelets in a given sample of blood.

**blood level** The amount of substance in a measured specimen of blood.

**bone marrow** A soft, spongy tissue in the cavity at the center of bones; made up of blood vessels, fat, and all-important hematopoietic (blood-forming) stem cells that develop into various cells in the blood. These include erythrocytes or red blood cells that carry oxygen, leukocytes or white blood cells that fight infection, and platelets that

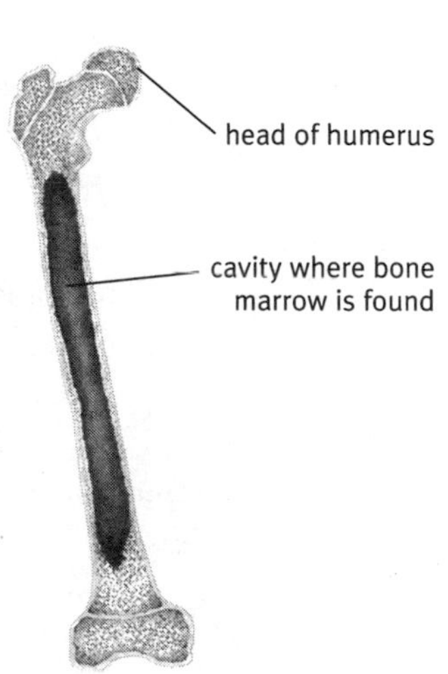

take part in blood clotting. Bone marrow injury (toxicity) is a common adverse side effect of most chemotherapy and radiation therapy.

**bone marrow transplant** A technique to graft bone marrow as a source of hematopoietic (blood-forming) stem cells, which are the precursors of white blood cells, red blood cells, and platelets. The technique is used to replace bone marrow destroyed by high-dose chemotherapy and/or whole-body irradiation. It is used to treat leukemia and lymphomas. Although previously used to treat patients with advanced breast cancer, its value in this disease is not certain at this time. Bone marrow previously harvested from the patient (autologous graft) or a genetically similar individual (allogeneic graft) is given intravenously, similar to a blood transfusion. A bone marrow transplant is a complex, lengthy, expensive procedure that is available only in cancer treatment centers. Stem cells can also be obtained from blood and can be used as a source for transplant cells. *See also* Stem Cell Transplant.

**bone scan** An imaging study of the skeleton, which is easily done and widely available, used to detect cancers that originate in, or have metastasized (spread) to, bone. A small amount of a radioisotope (technetium-99) is given intravenously, after which the body is surveyed (scanned) by a sensing device that detects gamma radiation. Areas of radiation (hot-spots) not only indicate cancer, but also many nonmalignant conditions, including benign tumor, healed fractures, arthritis.

**bone survey (skeletal)** An x-ray of all the bones of the body. It is often done when looking for cancer that has spread to the bone.

**bowel** *See* Intestine.

**Bowen's disease** A noninvasive skin cancer (in situ) of older people that appears as a raised brown or pink, sharply outlined, scaly growth on non sun-exposed areas (face, neck, arms, legs). Although easily cured by surgery, it is of concern because 80% of people with this tumor have another completely unrelated cancer. People with Bowen's disease should have a thorough physical examination and appropriate laboratory and other studies to detect a possible underlying malignancy of internal organs. *See also* Skin Cancer (pages 199–201); Squamous Cell Carcinoma.

**BPH** *See* Benign Prostatic Hypertrophy.

**brachytherapy** A radiation therapy technique in which the radiation source is contained within the body. It is either temporarily placed in a body opening (vagina, anus) adjacent to a cancer, or permanently or temporarily implanted in or next to a tumor. Brachytherapy is used much less often than external beam radiation (teletherapy) in which the radiation source (linear accelerator, cobalt generator) is located outside the body. It has been used more frequently in the treatment of cancer of the prostate gland in men. *See* Afterloading; Radiation Therapy.

**brain scan** An imaging method used to find anything abnormal in the brain, including brain cancer and cancer that has spread to the brain. A radioactive substance is injected into a vein and the images taken will show where radioactivity accumulates, indicating an abnormality. Brain scans of this type have been largely replaced by MRI and CT scans.

**BRCA** Two breast cancer genes, BRCA1 and BRCA2, which when defective, undergo mutation and are passed on to relatives sometimes causing female breast and ovarian cancers (BRCA1); and female and male breast cancers and in ovarian cancers (BRCA2). The defective BRCA gene is responsible for approximately 6% to 7% of breast cancers in women. Women with either of these gene mutations have a 40% to 80% lifetime risk of developing cancer. It is very important to follow through with screening and appropriate medical care and consultation. A blood test may be available in the future that will predict the few individuals with this gene who are at risk for breast and ovarian cancers. *See also* Appendix for Cancer Detection Guidelines; Breast Cancer (pages 159–161).

**breakthrough pain** A brief and often severe flare of pain that occurs even though a person may be taking pain medicine regularly for persistent pain (continuous pain that is present for long periods of time). It is called breakthrough pain because it is pain that "breaks through" a regular pain medicine schedule.

**breast augmentation** Surgery to increase the size of the breast. *See also* Breast Implant; Mammoplasty.

**breast conservation therapy** Surgery to remove a breast cancer and a small amount of benign tissue around the cancer without removing any other part of the breast. The lymph nodes under the arm may also be removed, and radiation therapy is often given after the surgery. *See also* Breast Cancer (pages 159–161).

**breast implant** A sac used to increase breast size or restore the contour of a breast after mastectomy. The sac is filled with silicone gel or sterile salt water. *See also* Breast Cancer (pages 159–161); Mastectomy.

**breast reconstruction** Surgery that rebuilds the breast contour after mastectomy. A breast implant or the woman's own tissue is used. Reconstruction can be done at the time of mastectomy or at a later time. *See also* Breast Cancer (pages 159–161); Mammoplasty; Mastectomy.

**breast self-examination (BSE)** A method of checking one's own breasts for lumps or suspicious changes. *See* Appendix for Cancer Detection Guidelines.

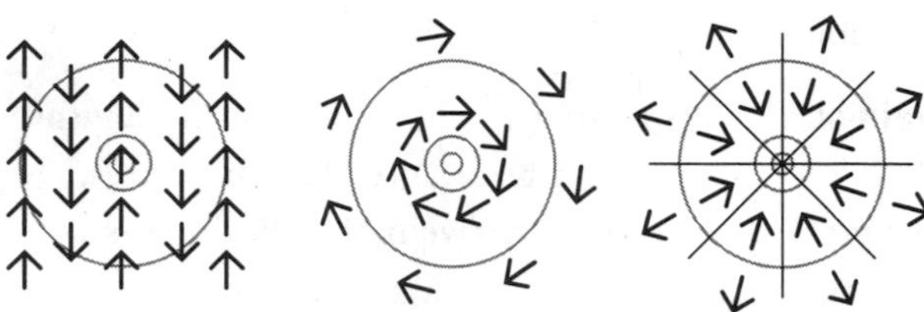

When performing a breast self-examination, move around the breast area in a circular, up and down line, or wedge pattern. Be sure to do it in the same way every time, check the entire breast area, and remember how your breast feels from month to month.

**Breslow microstaging** A technique for staging skin melanoma, which measures tumor thickness. It is considered more accurate than the Clark level staging method that determines depth of tumor growth. Used together, these two methods give an accurate estimation of how melanoma will behave, and help determine how it should be treated. *See also* Clark Level.

**bronchoalveolar cancer** An uncommon variety of non-small cell lung cancer (NSCLC); a type of adenocarcinoma. Occasionally, tumor spread throughout both lungs (as seen on chest x-ray) can be confused with pneumonia. *See also* Lung Cancer (pages 180–182); Non-Small Cell Lung Cancer.

**bronchogenic cancer** *See* Lung Cancer (pages 180–182).

**bronchoscope** A lighted, flexible, magnifying instrument used to examine and biopsy lesions or infections in the trachea or windpipe and large air passages (bronchi). It can also be used to remove foreign objects from the windpipe that may have been accidentally inhaled.

**bronchoscopy** A procedure using a bronchoscope; most often done under local anesthesia. It is invaluable for diagnosing lung disease, and determining the extent (stage) of lung cancer. *See also* Lung Cancer (pages 180–182).

**BSE** *See* Breast Self-Examination.

**BUN** Blood urea nitrogen is an indication of kidney function. The test measures the amount of urea, the end product of nitrogen metabolism in mammals, formed in the liver and removed in urine. Increased BUN occurs in kidney disease, urinary obstruction, and occasionally in gastrointestinal bleeding.

℞ **bupropion hydrochloride** Also known by the trade name Wellbutrin®, this drug is an aminoketone antidepressant used to relieve depression. It is also prescribed under the trade name Zyban®, a smoking cessation aid.

**Burkitt's lymphoma** An aggressive variety of non-Hodgkin's lymphoma, most often seen in children. Untreated, it is likely to cause death in a matter of weeks; however, it is curable in some cases. In Africa, it is a very common malignancy that causes extreme swelling of the jaw and face; but in the United States, it usually affects internal organs and causes an abdominal mass or lump. *See also* Non-Hodgkin's Lymphoma (pages 188–190).

Rx **BuSpar®** *See* Buspirone Hydrochloride.

Rx **buspirone hydrochloride** Also known by the trade name BuSpar®, this drug belongs to a group of drugs known as anxiolytic agents used to treat anxiety.

Rx **busulfan** Also known by the trade name Myleran®, this drug belongs to a group of drugs known as alkylating agents. It is used in the treatment of several types of cancer, including myelogenous leukemia, primarily in bone marrow and stem cell transplantation.

# C

**CA** The abbreviation for cancer, often confused with Ca, the chemical symbol for calcium.

**CA 15-3** Cancer antigen 15-3 is a tumor marker used as a blood test for breast cancer, which also may be positive in noncancerous fibrocystic breast disease. Used together with another tumor marker, carcinoembryonic antigen, CA 15-3 may indicate breast cancer that recurs after treatment. However, it is not practical to use this test on a routine basis for the early detection of recurrence after primary breast cancer therapy since it has not been demonstrated to change the overall course of the disease once it recurs at distant sites. *See also* Breast Cancer (pages 159–161); Tumor Marker.

**CA 19-9** Cancer antigen 19-9 is a tumor marker in blood used as a test for evaluating cancer of the pancreas. A pretreatment increase in the marker indicates advanced stages of pancreatic cancer and a poorer outcome. An increase in CA 19-9 following surgery may be the first indication of recurrent cancer. *See* Tumor Marker.

**CA 125** Cancer antigen 125 is a tumor marker in blood signaling epithelial ovarian carcinoma, the most common variety of ovarian cancer. Because 80% of women with advanced cancer of the ovary have increased levels of CA 125, the test is considered useful for diagnosing pelvic tumors. It is also used to identify women with either persistent or recurrent ovarian cancer following treatment. *See also* Ovarian Cancer (pages 190–191); Tumor Marker.

**cachexia** Weight loss and lessening of fat and muscle that accompanies advanced cancer, even with adequate nutrition. It is possibly due to substances released from the malignancy that causes the body to lose fat and protein. *See also* Paraneoplastic Syndrome.

**calcifications** Tiny calcium deposits within the breast, singly or in clusters, usually found by mammography. These are also called microcalcifications. They are a sign of change within the breast that may need to be followed by more mammograms or by a biopsy. Calcifications may be caused by benign breast conditions or by breast cancer.

**calcitonin** The hormone from thyroid, parathyroid, and thymus glands, which reduces the level of calcium in blood; used as a tumor marker for medullary thyroid cancer (MTC). It identifies MTC that recurs after surgery and C cell hyperplasia, the premalignant condition in families prone to develop medullary cancer. Calcitonin from animal sources is used to treat hypercalcemia (increased calcium in the blood) often caused by breast, prostate, and other cancers spread to bone. *See also* Tumor Marker.

**calcium** The major mineral component of the body, essential for growth of teeth and bone, which also exists outside the skeleton in cells and blood. It is responsible for such diverse functions as blood clotting, nerve transmission, and regulation of heartbeat. Hypercalcemia (an increased calcium level in the blood), often seen in cancer involving bone, is considered a medical emergency.

**CAM 17.1** A newly recognized tumor marker in blood that is more specific for pancreatic cancer than the marker CA 19-9. *See* Tumor Marker.

℞ **Campath®** *See* Alemtuzumab.

℞ **camphorated opium tincture** Also known by the trade name Paregoric®, this drug is an opioid antidiarrheal agent.

℞ **Camptosar®** *See* Irinotecan.

**cancer** Although usually thought of as a single disease, cancer encompasses almost 100 disorders caused by some 300 different growths. Cancer is known by other terms including malignancy, meaning that without treatment it will eventually cause death, and neoplasm, indicating new growth. Tumor is Latin for swelling. "Solid tumor" is used to describe cancer other than leukemia, lymphoma, and Hodgkin's disease.

Cancer may be thought of as the unchecked growth of out-of-control cells. Normal cells, the microscopic building blocks of all living things, have a definite life span and ultimately undergo apoptosis (stop reproducing and die) when removed from the body and grown artificially in the laboratory in tissue culture. However, cancer cells grown under similar laboratory conditions are immortal and continue to reproduce if supplied with nutrients and oxygen. The same is true for cancer cells in the body.

Although cancers differ from benign (noncancerous) tumors in many ways, the two most obvious differences are their ability to invade (grow into) and destroy adjacent normal body structures and organs, and to spread or metastasize to lymph nodes and other organs. *See* Highlights section for more detailed information on specific cancers.

**cancer cell** A cell that divides and reproduces abnormally and can spread throughout the body.

**cancer family syndrome** A condition in which certain cancers repeatedly occur in a family. The Lynch cancer syndrome is present when one or more generations have colorectal cancers not associated with multiple intestinal polyps (Lynch type I); or colorectal, endometrial, ovarian, and (rarely) stomach and other cancers (Lynch type II). The Li-Fraumeni or SBLA syndrome occurs when a family has repeated malignancies including sarcoma, breast cancer, bone cancer, brain tumor, leukemia, lung cancer, laryngeal cancer, and adrenal gland tumors. Also called familial cancer syndrome.

**cancer susceptibility genes** Genes (the basic unit of heredity) inherited from one's parents that greatly increase the risk of a person developing cancer. Approximately 5% to 15% of all cancers are caused by these genes.

**cancerous** Relating to cancer. *See also* Malignant.

***Candida*** A yeast-like fungus that often causes infections (candidiasis) in people with low numbers of white blood cells (most often from cancer chemotherapy) who have received antibiotics to prevent bacterial infection. Candidiasis causes problems including painful mouth ulcers and severe and even fatal infections of esophagus, liver, and lungs. Treatment is with intravenous antifungal medication such as amphotericin B and with oral medication including ketoconazole.

℞ **capecitabine** Also known by the trade name Xeloda®, this is an antimetabolite type of chemotherapy drug used for widespread breast and colon cancer. Although it is converted by enzymes in a tumor to the anticancer drug fluorouracil (5-FU), it causes less bone marrow injury and hair loss than does 5-FU. Side effects include severe diarrhea, nausea, vomiting, pain, and swelling of hands and feet.

**capsule formation** Scar tissue that may form around a breast implant (or other type of implant) as the body reacts to the foreign object. Sometimes called a contracture.

℞ **carbenicillin indanyl sodium** Also known by the trade names Geocillin® and Geopen®, this drug is an antibiotic that belongs to a group of drugs known as extended-spectrum penicillins.

℞ **carboplatin** Also known by the trade name Paraplatin®, this chemotherapy drug is similar to cisplatin, but with milder and better-tolerated adverse side effects. It is used primarily as treatment of ovarian cancer. Carboplatin can be given either intravenously or injected inside the peritoneal cavity (abdomen). Nausea and vomiting are more easily controlled than are similar side effects associated with cisplatin. And nephrotoxicity (injury to the kidney), a common adverse effect of cisplatin, is uncommon with the use of this drug.

**carcinoembryonic antigen (CEA)** A tumor marker in blood used as a test for colon and rectal cancers and for other malignancies including breast cancer. For people who have undergone surgery for colorectal cancer, an elevated CEA level in blood may indicate persistent or recurrent tumor. Increased blood levels of CEA also occur in cigarette smokers with no evidence of cancer.

**carcinogen** Any substance, agent, or condition that causes cancer. Among these causative factors are: environmental—radiation (radon, solar, x-rays), chemical compounds (aniline dye, asbestos); lifestyle—alcohol abuse, tobacco abuse (cigarettes, snuff); dietary—contaminants (aflatoxin), preservatives (nitrate-nitrite); infection—viral (genital herpes, hepatitis, HIV).

**carcinoid** A rare, unusual, slow growing tumor of the gastrointestinal (GI) tract or the lungs that produces the hormone serotonin. The tumor is considered malignant only if it has spread to lymph nodes or other organs, which usually occurs only with large tumors. Carcinoids in the liver or lung that release large amounts of serotonin can cause the carcinoid syndrome, a combination of symptoms and lesions that includes wheezing, reddening and flushing (warming) of neck and face, diarrhea, and scarring of the heart. The severity of the syndrome depends on the size and number of tumors producing serotonin. The diagnosis of carcinoid tumor depends upon the presence of either serotonin or 5-hydroxyindoleacetic acid (5-HIAA) derived from serotonin and measured in a urine sample collected over a 24-hour period. Most carcinoids occur in the appendix and are discovered (and cured) by appendectomy. However, tumors in the rectum and small intestine, unless very small, usually require removal of adjacent lymph nodes as well as a portion of the intestine. Tumor(s) spread to the liver that do not cause the carcinoid syndrome usually do not need treatment. Severe flushing and diarrhea are often controlled by octreotide (Sandostatin®), a drug that counteracts serotonin. If octreotide is not successful, chemotherapy drugs (doxorubicin, dacarbazine) can be injected into the hepatic artery (artery to the liver) followed by a small piece of absorbable sponge (Gelfoam) to block the flow of blood through the artery and control symptoms.

**carcinoma** The most common type of cancer in adults, which includes skin, lung, prostate, colorectal, and ovarian tumors. Although they differ in many ways, all carcinomas arise in epithelium, tissue that acts variously to cover the body (skin), line internal organs (mucosa), and release hormones and other substances (glands). Carcinomas that form glands are called adenocarcinomas; and those that produce keratin, a protein material normally found in skin, hair, and nails, are called squamous cell carcinomas. Rapidly growing tumors that do not resemble either adenocarcinomas or squamous carcinomas are called undifferentiated carcinomas. *See also* Cancer.

**carcinoma in situ** The earliest stage of carcinoma, before it becomes invasive and penetrates or invades underlying tissue. It is most often used to describe early skin, breast, cervical, and bladder cancers, and early melanoma. These preinvasive tumors do not cause metastasis, and with proper treatment all are curable. Untreated, they can progress to invasive cancer with the potential to metastasize (spread). They may be removed surgically or eradicated using electrocautery (electric current), cryotherapy (freezing), laser, and chemotherapy applied directly. *See also* Preinvasive Cancer.

**cardiomyopathy** Disease of the heart muscle, which in cancer patients can be caused by radiation therapy to the chest and by anticancer drug therapy, especially doxorubicin and trastuzumab. Usual problems are irregular heartbeat and heart failure (failure of the heart to pump blood efficiently), which may not appear until months following treatment. Limiting the dose of chemotherapy and shielding the heart from radiation prevents or lessens cardiac injury. The drug dexrazoxane, given for several weeks following doxorubicin therapy, reduces the severity of cardiomyopathy in both children and adults.

**carmustine** *See* Nitrosourea.

**carotid body tumor** A usually benign tumor of the carotid body; a small structure in each side of the neck attached to a carotid artery. These small organs control rate and depth of breathing in response to changes in blood: lack of oxygen, an excess of carbon dioxide, and increased acidity (low pH). Although seldom malignant, these tumors can enlarge and interfere with breathing and blood flow to the brain. Surgical removal is usual, but radiation therapy may be used. *See* Paraganglioma, Neuroendocrine Tumor.

**cartilage** Firm, flexible tissue without a blood supply that covers the ends of bones and gives support to the larynx, nose, and ears. Cartilage gives rise to both benign tumors (chondroma) and cancer (chondrosarcoma).

℞ **Casodex®** *See* Bicalutamide.

**castration** Removal of the ovaries (bilateral oophorectomy) or testicles (bilateral orchiectomy). The operation is used as hormone manipulation for treating advanced-stage cancers whose growth is stimulated by sex hormones: estrogen in females, and androgen in males. Although oophorectomy is seldom used for female breast cancer, orchiectomy is often used in prostate cancer and occasionally in male breast cancer. *See* Oophorectomy; Orchiectomy.

**cat eye reflex** *See* Leukocoria; Retinoblastoma.

**CAT scan** Also called CT; *See* Computed Tomography.

℞ **Catapres®** *See* Clonidine Hydrochloride.

**catecholamine** The hormones epinephrine and norepinephrine, which are produced by the central part of the adrenal gland (adrenal medulla), increase blood pressure, heart rate, and breathing rate. Excess catecholamine from pheochromocytoma, a rare, usually benign tumor of the adrenal medulla, causes intermittent or sustained, extremely severe, hypertension (high blood pressure) and sudden death.

**catheter** A thin, flexible tube which can be used to inject fluids into the body or to drain fluids from the body, such as a tube to drain urine. Catheters are also used in various diagnostic and treatment procedures, such as directing chemotherapy into the liver or treating blocked blood vessels in the heart.

**cavity** A hollow space in the body. The chest cavity contains the lungs, heart, and large blood vessels to the heart. The abdominal cavity, which contains the stomach, intestines, liver, and spleen, is continuous with the pelvic cavity (pelvis), which contains the rectum, bladder, and women's reproductive organs.

**CBC** *See* Complete Blood Count.

**C cell hyperplasia** A precancerous condition that gives rise to medullary carcinoma cancer, an uncommon variety of thyroid cancer that may be inherited in the multiple endocrine neoplasia (MEN) syndrome.

℞ **CCNU®** Trade name for lomustine. *See* Nitrosourea.

**CEA** *See* Carcinoembryonic Antigen.

℞ **Ceclor®** *See* Cefaclor.

**cecum** The first 3 to 4 inches of large intestine in the lower right side of the abdomen. Weakness due to anemia from unrecognized intestinal bleeding may be the first symptom of cecal cancer, which is becoming more common. *See also* Colorectal Cancer (pages 163–165).

℞ **cefaclor** Also known by the trade name Ceclor®, this drug is an antibiotic that belongs to a group of drugs known as cephalosporins.

℞ **cefamandole nafate** Also known by the trade name Mandol®, this drug is an antibiotic that belongs to a group of drugs known as cephalosporins.

℞ **cefazolin sodium** Also known by the trade names Kefzol® and Ancel®, this drug is an antibiotic that belongs to a group of drugs known as cephalosporins.

℞ **cefdinir** Also known by the trade name Omnicef®, it belongs to the general class of drugs known as cephalosporin broad spectrum antibiotics. Cefdinir prevents bacteria from making their cell walls and is active against some bacteria that are resistant to penicillins. It is used to treat pneumonia, worsening bronchitis, sinusistis, pharyngitis, and tonsillitis.

℞ **cefepime** Also known by the trade name Maxipime®, this antibiotic belongs to the class of drugs known as cephalosporins. It is used to treat infections of the respiratory and urinary tracts, skin, and abdomen. It is active against some bacteria that are resistant to other antibiotics.

℞ **cefixime** Also known by the trade name Suprax®, this drug is an antibiotic that belongs to a group of drugs known as cephalosporins.

℞ **cefotaxime sodium** Also known by the trade name Claforan®, this drug is an antibiotic that belongs to a group of drugs known as cephalosporins.

℞ **cefoxitin sodium** Also known by the trade name Mefoxin®, this drug is an antibiotic that belongs to a group of drugs known as cephalosporins.

℞ **ceftazidime** Also known by the trade names Fortaz®, Tazicef®, and Tazidime®, this drug is an antibiotic that belongs to a group of drugs known as cephalosporins.

℞ **ceftriaxone sodium** Also known by the trade name Rocephin®, this drug is an antibiotic that belongs to a group of drugs known as cephalosporins.

℞ **Celebrex®** *See* Celecoxib.

℞ **celecoxib** Also known by the trade name Celebrex®, this drug is used to reduce the number of colon and rectal polyps (adenomatous polyps) in people with familial adenomatous polyposis, who have hundreds or thousands of intestinal polyps that are likely to become cancerous unless removed. Initially approved to treat arthritis, it is being studied as a preventive medicine for all colorectal cancers.

**cell** The smallest bit of living matter able to survive by itself; the basic building block of all living things. Collections or layers of similar cells in plants and animals form tissue.

**cell cycle** A theoretical model illustrating how cells reproduce and proliferate (make exact copies of themselves). This model divides cellular proliferation into distinct periods: G0, Gap1 (G1), DNA synthesis (S), Gap2 (G2), and mitosis (M), and is used to explain how radiation and chemotherapy drugs affect cells during certain periods of cellular growth. Because cancer cells reproduce (cycle) faster than most normal cells (except for those in bone marrow), malignancies are more sensitive than normal tissue to the effects of chemotherapy and radiation therapy.

**central nervous system cancer** *See* Brain Tumor (pages 157–159).

Rx **cephradine** Also known by the trade names Anspor® and Velosef®, this drug is an antibiotic that belongs to a group of drugs known as cephalosporins.

**cerebellopontine angle tumor** *See* Acoustic Neuroma.

**cerebral edema** Accumulation of watery fluid in the brain that causes it to swell and increase pressure within the skull; often due to brain tumors and cancers that have spread to the brain. Cerebral edema can be fatal unless promptly treated, and drugs similar to cortisone (Decadron®) and mannitol that draws fluid from brain are often life-saving. *See also* Brain Tumor (pages 157–159).

**cerebrospinal fluid** Clear watery fluid produced in the brain, which surrounds both the brain and spinal cord. Examination of cerebrospinal fluid obtained by lumbar puncture (needle puncture of the spine) is used to diagnose disorders of the brain and spinal cord, such as hemorrhage and infection, but is seldom used to diagnose brain tumors. In some cases, anticancer drugs injected into spinal fluid are used to treat tumors of the brain and spinal cord.

Rx **Cerubidine®** *See* Daunorubicin.

**cervical** Relating to the cervix or lower, narrow portion of the uterus. *See also* Cervical Cancer (pages 161–163).

**cervix** The elongated, lower portion or neck of the uterus (womb) where it joins the birth canal or vagina. *See also* Appendix for Cancer Detection Guidelines; Cervical Cancer (pages 161–163).

**chemotherapy** Treatment with drugs that destroy cancer cells. Chemotherap is often used with surgery or radiation to treat cancer that has spread, that h come back (recurred), or that has a strong chance of recurring. The type of chemotherapy used depends on many factors, including the type of tumor, location, and stage of disease, age, health status, personal preferences, and other factors. *See also* Radiation Therapy; Surgical Therapy.

**childhood cancer** Although rare in children (8,600 new cases each year), cancer is second only to trauma (accidents) as the leading killer of children under age 15 in the United States, leading to about 1,500 deaths each year. However, 75% of pediatric cancer patients will survive 5 years or more. This is twice the number of children who survived cancer 25 years ago. Childhood cancers are not merely adult cancers that strike children. They are distinct malignancies that behave differently from those in older people and should be treated in children's cancer centers. Unlike common cancers in adults, those in children are rarely carcinomas and seldom, if ever, affect the lung, breast, prostate, and colon, commonly the sites of adult malignancies. In contrast to adult cancers, pediatric malignancies usually grow faster and are more affected by age and gender. As a rule, cancers in children respond more readily to drugs and radiation treatment than do those in adults, and advanced-stage pediatric malignancies are often more curable than are advanced-stage adult malignancies. Combined treatment with surgery, chemotherapy, and radiation generally is more successful in children than adults.

Although leukemia and lymphoma account for almost half of all childhood cancers, 70% to 90% of children with these malignancies live for at least 5 years after starting therapy. Of the pediatric solid cancers (malignancies other than leukemia, lymphoma, and Hodgkin's disease), brain tumors are the most common, followed by neuroblastoma, Wilms' tumor, bone and muscle sarcomas. Rhabdomyosarcoma is the most common soft tissue sarcoma in children. Retinoblastoma (cancer of the eye), although rare, accounts for 5% of childhood blindness.

Although the outlook for most pediatric cancer patients is favorable, those who survive must be followed closely throughout their lives. Except for those few who show varying degrees of brain damage from radiation therapy of childhood brain tumors, most adults who survive childhood cancers lead essentially normal lives. However, heart disease, and second malignancies having nothing to do with prior cancers occur earlier and more often among pediatric cancer survivors, due to long-term effects of chemotherapy and radiation. Also, some children will have growth problems.

*See also* Bone Cancer (pages 156–157); Leukemia (pages 176–178); Neuroblastoma (pages 187–188); Non-Hodgkin's Lymphoma (pages 188–190); Retinoblastoma (pages 196–197); Rhabdomyosarcoma; Wilms' Tumor (pages 212–213).

**chlorambucil** Also known by the trade name Leukeran®, this is an alkylating type of chemotherapy drug similar to nitrogen mustard. It is taken by mouth to treat chronic lymphocytic leukemia, lymphoma, and Hodgkin's disease. Its use is associated with an increased risk of developing acute myelogenous leukemia (AML).

**chlorpromazine** Also known by the trade name Thorazine®, this is a drug for treating nausea that is given by mouth, injection, or rectal suppository. Its main unwanted side effects include drowsiness and tardive dyskinesia (uncontrolled movements of the face and tongue).

**Cholac®** *See* Lactulose.

**cholangiocarcinoma** A rare type of liver cancer that arises in the bile ducts within the liver. *See* Bile Duct Cancer (pages 153–154).

**cholangitis** Inflammation of the bile ducts that collect and drain bile from the liver into the digestive tract. It is often related to obstruction from stones in the common bile, and infected bile; is known to accompany the inflammatory bowel disease known as chronic ulcerative colitis. Also, cholangitis can be caused when floxuridine (FUDR®), a drug used to treat cancer that has spread to the liver, is given over long periods through the hepatic artery to the liver (continuous intra-arterial infusion). In the Orient, inflammation of the bile ducts often is due to parasites (liver flukes) in bile ducts. Cholangitis is associated with bile duct cancer and with hepatobiliary (liver) cancer that arises in the liver. *See also* Bile Duct Cancer (pages 153–154); Liver Cancer (pages 178–179).

**cholecystectomy** Surgical removal of the gallbladder. *See also* Gallbladder Cancer (pages 168–170).

**choline magnesium trisalicylate** Also known by the trade name Trilisate®, this drug is a nonopioid analgesic that belongs to a group of drugs known as salicylates. It is also known as a nonsteroidal anti-inflammatory drug (NSAID), and is an alternative to aspirin in certain clinical situations such as aspirin sensitivity.

**chondrosarcoma** Any one of several cancers that arise in cartilage, the firm tissue without a blood supply, which covers the ends of bones in joints and gives internal support to the nose, ears, and larynx. This type of bone cancer occurs most often in the pelvis, thigh, upper arm, breastbone, and shoulder blade, in middle age and older adults. It arises either as a new (*de novo*) growth or from a pre-existing benign tumor (chondroma).

**chorioadenoma destruens** An hydatidiform mole (tumorous growth of tissue from the placenta or afterbirth, tissue that connects the fetus and mother) with a tendency to invade surrounding tissue, but which very seldom metastasizes (spreads) elsewhere. Also called invasive mole.

**choriocarcinoma** An uncommon cancer of the afterbirth or placenta (tissue that joins the fetus and mother), which spreads early to distant organs, including lung, vagina, brain, and liver. It occurs in the uterus during pregnancy and can also affect the ovary of non-pregnant females, the testis of males, and the center of the chest or mediastinum, most often in young men. This malignant tumor produces the hormone beta human chorionic gonadotropin (β-hCG), which is used as a tumor marker to reflect both response to treatment and to indicate recurrence after treatment.

**chromosome** Any one of 46 microscopic structures in the nucleus (rounded mass of material in the center of every human cell). Each chromosome carries thousands of genes (units that transmit hereditary information responsible for cell character and growth). The X and Y (sex chromosomes) are the ones that determine the gender of an individual: XX for female, XY for male. Abnormal chromosomes, which in some cases appear responsible for normal cells becoming cancerous, are used to identify certain cancers and to predict their behavior; for instance, the Philadelphia chromosome (Ph1) in white blood cells in chronic myelocytic leukemia and acute lymphoblastic leukemia. *See also* DNA; Philadelphia Chromosome.

**chronic** Any medical condition that persists; for biomedical statistical purposes any problem that lasts for 3 or more months. It implies a condition that is less severe than one of acute or sudden onset.

℞ **cidofovir** Also known by the trade name Vistide®, this drug belongs to a group of drugs known as antiviral agents. It is used in the treatment of a particular eye infection (cytomegalovirus retinitis), and has potentially severe adverse effects on kidney function.

℞ **Cipro®** *See* Ciprofloxacin.

℞ **ciprofloxacin** Also known by the trade name Cipro®, this drug is an antibiotic that belongs to a group of drugs known as fluoroquinolones.

**cirrhosis** Progressive liver disease that causes the liver to scar and shrink in size; often the forerunner of hepatocellular cancer or hepatoma, a type of liver cancer that originates in liver cells. Among its many causes are alcohol abuse, hepatitis (a chronic viral infection), certain inherited metabolic diseases, and exposure to industrial chemicals, notably carbon tetrachloride. *See also* Liver Cancer (pages 178–179).

℞ **cisplatin** Also known as cis-platinum (Platinol®), this chemotherapy drug is classified as a heavy-metal type of alkylating agent. It is widely used to treat a variety of cancers, with the greatest impact on ovarian and testicular tumors. Although kidney injury is the most severe unwanted side effect of the compound, severe nausea is its most noticeable problem.

℞ **cis-platinum** *See* Cisplatin.

**citrovorum factor** *See* Leucovorin.

℞ **Citrucel®** *See* Methylcellulose.

℞ **cladribine** Also known by the trade name Leustatin®, this drug belongs to a group of drugs known as antimetabolites. It is used in the treatment of several types of cancer, including hairy cell leukemia.

℞ **Claforan®** *See* Cefotaxime Sodium.

**Clark level** Used in skin (cutaneous) melanoma to delineate the level of deepening tumor penetration and to define the stage or extent of disease. Microscopic study of the cancer assigns different levels (Level I-V) based upon growth of tumor into different layers of skin and underlying, fatty subcutaneous tissue. The outlook for melanoma worsens with successive involvement of each level. *See also* Breslow Microstaging.

**clear cell vaginal cancer** An unusual cancer of the vagina of older girls and young women whose mothers received diethylstilbestrol, a synthetic hormone with estrogen-like effects, prescribed between 1940 and 1971 to prevent miscarriage. It most often affects girls 15 to 22 years of age. *See also* Vaginal Cancer (pages 209–211).

℞ **Cleocin®** *See* Clindamycin Phosphate.

℞ **clindamycin phosphate** Also known by the trade name Cleocin®, this drug is an antibiotic that belongs to a group of drugs known as antibacterial agents.

**clinical trial** A human test or investigation, often carried out on cancer patients to study the safety and benefits of potential new treatment methods. These carefully done studies are conducted with the complete understanding and cooperation of those who volunteer to take part. Investigations often involve one of three phases:

*Phase 1:* Involves advanced-cancer patients who have failed usual treatment; to determine optimal dose, preferred delivery method (intravenous, oral), and adverse side effects.

*Phase 2:* Done on people with advanced cancer that can be measured or evaluated by physical, laboratory, x-rays or other imaging studies; to determine if the cancer will respond to therapy evaluated in Phase I studies.

*Phase 3:* Used to compare new treatment with a known method. The most accurate study is the double-blind study in which neither patient nor investigator knows what therapy the patient is receiving until the study is concluded, which may take many years.

℞ **clonazepam** Also known by the trade name Klonopin®, this drug belongs to a group of drugs known as benzodiazepines. It is used for the treatment of anxiety and panic disorder.

℞ **clonidine hydrochloride** Also known by the trade names Duraclon® and Catapres®, this drug belongs to a group of drugs known as centrally acting alpha-adrenergic agonists. It is most commonly used for the treatment of hypertension. It is also injected into the spinal cord as an infusion for the treatment of severe pain. Its major side effect is severe low blood pressure.

**clotting time** A laboratory study that measures the time it takes a blood sample to clot or coagulate. Used to regulate the dose of heparin, an anticoagulant drug that prolongs blood clotting. *See also* Heparin.

**cobalt therapy** Radiation therapy that uses radioactive cobalt as the source of x-rays. Once widely used in this country to treat cancer, it has largely been replaced by an electrical device, the linear accelerator. *See also* Radiation Therapy.

℞ **codeine** This drug is an opioid analgesic. It is similar to morphine, but less potent. It is used as a pain reliever for mild to moderate pain, frequently in combination with acetaminophen.

**colectomy** Complete or partial removal of the colon; used to treat colon and rectal (colorectal) cancer. May also be used in the treatment of some nonmalignant diseases, such as ulcerative colitis. *See also* Colorectal Cancer (pages 163–165).

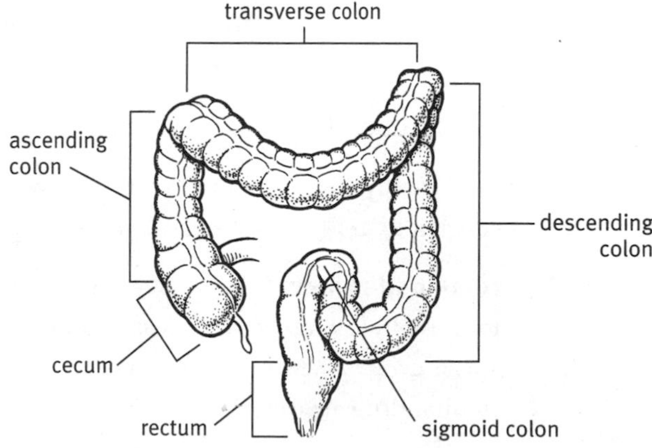


**colo-** Pertaining to the colon, which together with the rectum comprises the large intestine.

**colon** The major portion of the large intestine, arbitrarily divided into five parts: cecum, right (ascending), transverse, left (descending), and sigmoid. *See also* Colorectal Cancer (pages 163–165); Intestine.

**colonoscope** A long, flexible, lighted magnifying instrument often connected to a television monitor; used to examine, biopsy, and remove growths from the large intestine or colon. *See also* Colorectal Cancer (pages 163–165).

**colonoscopy** The procedure using a colonoscope introduced through the anus. It is done under sedation, and does not require hospitalization. Preparation for the procedure includes laxatives and occasionally enemas to be certain the colon surface is as clean as possible. In many instances, colonoscopy has replaced barium enema as the preferred method for screening and diagnosing colon and rectal cancers. It is also used to find recurrent cancer in the colon after colon surgery. *See also* Colorectal Cancer (pages 163–165).

**colony stimulating factor** *See* Cytokine.

**colorectal** Relating to the colon and rectum, or to the entire bowel (large intestine).

**colostomy** A stoma (artificial opening), either temporary or permanent, created surgically between the colon and skin to divert bowel movements. When colorectal cancer causes obstruction, a temporary colostomy is needed before the colon can be removed. A permanent colostomy is necessary following abdominoperineal resection and for cancer blocking the large intestine that cannot be removed. The need for a bag (appliance) to contain stool depends on the site in the colon where the colostomy is done. In some individuals with a sigmoid colostomy following removal of the rectum, an early morning enema (irrigation) and avoidance of foods that cause loose stool enables them to do well without a colostomy bag. After receiving dietary information and instructions from a stomal therapist, almost all "colostomates" are able to lead normal, active lives. *See also* Stoma.

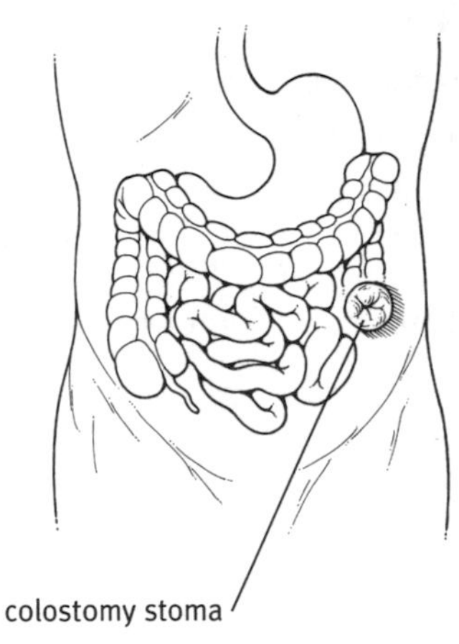


**colposcope** A lighted magnifying instrument to examine the vagina and cervix.

**colposcopy** Examination using a colposcope; often advised after a Pap test shows suspicious cells. It is a simple, painless procedure done in a physician's office.

**combination hormone therapy** Complete blockage of androgen production that may include orchiectomy (castration) or LHRH analogs as well as the use of antiandrogens. Also called total hormonal ablation; total androgen blockade; total androgen ablation.

**comedo carcinoma** A very early-stage breast cancer; the most aggressive variety of ductal carcinoma in situ (DCIS); so-called because the tumor filling small milk ducts can be squeezed out similar to a comedo (blackhead).

℞ **Compazine®** *See* Prochlorperazine.

**complementary therapy** A therapy used in addition to standard therapy. Some complementary therapies may relieve certain symptoms of cancer, relieve side effects of cancer therapy, or improve a patient's sense of well being.

**complete blood count (CBC)** A common laboratory blood test that determines type and number of white blood cells, number and quality of red blood cells, and number of platelets in a specimen of blood. The CBC is used to monitor the toxic effects that many chemotherapy drugs have on bone marrow in order to regulate their dose.

**computed tomography (CT)** An imaging technique that uses computer analysis to generate multiple cross-sectional x-ray pictures of the body. CT, also known as CAT scan, has revolutionized medical diagnostic studies and is invaluable in diagnosing and staging internal cancers. *See also* Imaging Study.

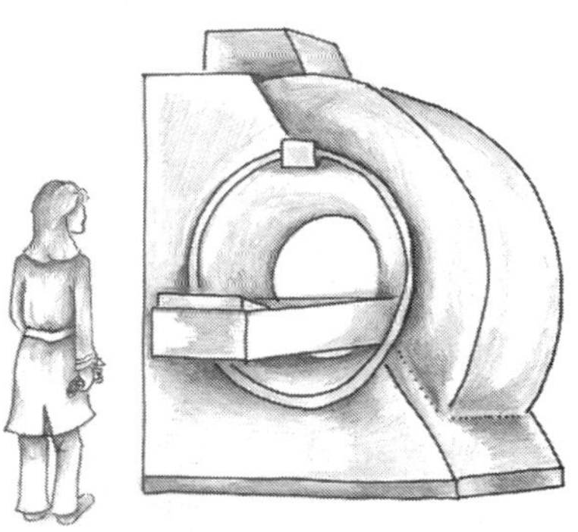

CT scanner

**conformal proton beam irradiation therapy** A technique using proton beams to deliver radiation to cancer cells. Protons are parts of atoms that cause little damage to tissue they pass through but are very effective in killing cells at the end of their path. *See also* Radiation Therapy.

**contracture** A capsule or shell of dense scar-like tissue that may form around a breast implant. *See also* Breast Implant; Capsule Formation.

**core needle biopsy** A biopsy procedure that uses a large-bore needle, such as the Trucut needle, to obtain a tissue sample for diagnosing cancer and other diseases. It is used to biopsy the prostate gland, liver, and breast, and is valuable because it provides a tissue sample the diameter of a toothpick for analysis. *See also* Biopsy.

**corticosteroid** A hormone produced by the cortex (outer layer) of the adrenal gland. It is categorized as mineralcorticoid, which regulates the amount of sodium, potassium, and water in the blood; glucocorticoid, the most potent corticosteroid, which affects the metabolism of fat, protein, and carbohydrate, and lessens inflammation (swelling, heat, redness, pain); and androgen, which affects development of masculine characteristics. *See also* Cortisone; Hydrocortisone.

**cortisol** A hormone produced by the adrenal gland. Overproduction of cortisol leads to Cushing's Syndrome. *See also* Cortisone; Cushing's Syndrome.

℞ **cortisone** Also known as hydrocortisone, this synthetic form of cortisol is more potent than the cortisol produced by the adrenal gland. These drugs are used to treat a variety of conditions including cancer. *See also* Cortisol.

℞ **co-trimoxazole (trimethoprim and sulfamethoxazole)** Also known by the trade name Bactrim®, this drug combination contains two antibiotics belonging to the sulfonamide group. It is particularly useful in the treatment of uncomplicated urinary tract infection, but is also used in the treatment and prevention of infections in patients infected with HIV (the virus that causes AIDS).

℞ **Coumadin®** *See* Warfarin.

**craniotomy** An operation to open the cranium (skull). It exposes the brain to permit surgeries on the brain, such as those to remove tumors, treat blood vessel enlargements (aneurysms), and relieve intracranial pressure (pressure in the skull) due to brain tumors that cannot be removed.

**creatinine** A chemical compound produced in muscle, filtered from blood by the kidneys, and eliminated in urine. It is used as a test of kidney function. The level of creatinine in a blood sample indicates the degree of renal (kidney) failure.

**Crohn's disease** A disease of unknown origin that causes severe intestinal inflammation (a reaction of tissue that includes swelling, warmth, pain). It usually affects the small intestine (duodenum, jejunum, ileum); and similar to the other inflammatory colon disease, ulcerative colitis, it can affect the colon and rectum. Crohn's disease of the small bowel increases the likelihood of small intestine cancer, and of the large bowel somewhat increases the risk of colorectal cancer. Also called regional enteritis or granulomatous colitis. *See also* Inflammatory Bowel Disease; Ulcerative Colitis.

**cryotherapy** Cancer treatment using extreme cold to destroy a tumor. Liquid nitrogen applied to bone is used for both sarcoma (bone cancer) and metastases (spread) to bone, and applied to skin is used for small skin cancers other than melanoma. More recently, metal probes cooled to subzero temperatures have been used to treat prostate and liver cancers.

**cryptorchidism** Failure of one or both testicles (testes) to descend into the scrotum (sac) beneath the penis, which normally takes place before birth. Cryptorchidism is the only factor known to increase the risk of testicular cancer; however, it is responsible for only about 10% of these malignancies. Also called cryptorchism.

**cryptorchism** *See* Cryptorchidism.

**CT** *See* Computed Tomography.

**C-Trak® probe** An instrument to detect and measure gamma radiation; used to identify the lymph node(s) (sentinel node) closest to a melanoma of the skin and likely to be the first involved with metastasis (spread). Melanoma cells in the sentinel node indicate the need for removal of all adjacent (regional) nodes. The device is being investigated to identify the sentinel node(s) in breast cancer.

**Cushing's disease** *See* Cushing's Syndrome.

**Cushing's syndrome** An endocrine disorder characterized by obesity of the trunk, a round (moon-shaped) face, abdominal striae (stretch marks), osteoporosis (bone thinning), and diabetes. It results from excess cortisol, a potent hormone that is produced in the outer layer, or cortex, of the adrenal glands. Cushing's syndrome is caused by both cancerous and noncancerous cortisol-producing tumors of the adrenal cortex and by a variety of other malignant tumors, especially small cell lung cancer that produces adrenocorticotropic hormone (ACTH), which stimulates the adrenal cortex. Cushing's disease is the syndrome caused by basophil adenoma (a nonmalignant tumor) of the pituitary gland at the base (undersurface) of the brain.

℞ **cyclophosphamide** Also known by the trade name Cytoxan®, this is an antimetabolite-type cancer chemotherapy drug given by mouth or injection. It is used in the chemotherapy of many different malignancies, especially breast cancer. Adverse side effects include injury to bone marrow and bladder irritation (cystitis).

**cyst** Any benign (noncancerous), bag-like growth or sac that contains fluid or soft material. Fluid-filled breast cysts due to fibrocystic changes are the most common cause of breast lumps. Various types commonly affect the skin (sebaceous cyst), thyroid, pancreas, liver, and ovaries.

**cystectomy** Partial or complete surgical removal of the urinary bladder, used to treat advanced-stage bladder cancer and other pelvic cancers involving the bladder. Total cystectomy requires an artificial bladder, such as the ileal bladder, to collect and hold urine. *See also* Bladder Cancer (pages 154–156).

**cystoscope** A lighted, tubular magnifying instrument passed through the urethra to examine the interior of the bladder. *See also* Bladder Cancer (pages 154–156).

**cystoscopy** The procedure using a cystoscope to visualize the interior of the bladder and biopsy large tumors and remove smaller growths by snaring, or destroying them with electrocautery (electric current). *See also* Bladder Cancer (pages 154–156).

Rx **cytarabine (cytosine arabinoside)** Also known by the trade name Cytosar-U®, this drug belongs to a group of drugs known as antimetabolites. It is used in the treatment of several types of cancer, including acute leukemia.

**cytokine** Any one of a variety of proteins produced in very minute amounts by certain white blood cells (lymphocytes and monocytes), which control the intensity and duration of the body's immune (protective) mechanism and interaction between cells. Cytokines being studied extensively as anticancer agents include: interleukins, interferons, and tumor necrosis factors. Colony-stimulating factors, cytokines that stimulate the bone marrow, are used to restore blood cells following a stem cell transplant.

**cytology** The microscopic study of cell samples (from urine, sputum, cyst contents, breast drainage) for the presence of cancer cells. The specimens are obtained by Pap test, fine needle aspiration biopsy, or other procedures.

**cytoreductive surgery** This is a surgical procedure intended to remove as much malignant tumor as possible from the abdomen to enable chemotherapy to be more effective. It is used for advanced and recurrent ovarian cancer, fallopian tube cancer, and peritoneal cancer. Also called debulking.

Rx **Cytosar-U®** *See* Cytarabine (Cytosine Arabinoside).

**cytotoxic** Anything injurious or poisonous to cells. Because many drugs used in cancer chemotherapy are cytotoxic to normal as well as malignant cells, the dose of these agents is limited by their effect on normal cells, especially bone marrow.

Rx **Cytovene®** *See* Ganciclovir.

Rx **Cytoxan®** *See* Cyclophosphamide.

# D

Rx **dacarbazine** Also known by the trade name DTIC-Dome®, this is a chemotherapy drug that acts similar to an alkylating agent. It is used in the treatment of several types of cancer, including Hodgkin's disease and melanoma.

℞ **dactinomycin** Also known by the trade name Actinomycin D®, this is an anti-tumor antibiotic used in chemotherapy of a variety of childhood cancers, sarcomas, and melanoma. Injury to bone marrow resulting in a reduced number of white blood cell is a common adverse side effect, as are nausea and vomiting. If this medication extravasates (leaks from a vein into the surrounding tissue), it can result in severe pain, swelling, and skin damage.

℞ **Daunomycin®** *See* Daunorubicin.

℞ **daunorubicin** Also known by the trade names Cerubidine®, Daunomycin®, and Rubidomycin®, this drug belongs to a group of drugs known as anthracycline antibiotics. It is used to treat several types of cancer, including acute myelocytic leukemia.

℞ **daunorubicin citrate liposome injection** Also known by the trade name Dauno-Xome®, this drug belongs to a group of drugs known as anthracycline antibiotics that are lipid encapsulated. It is used to treat several types of cancer, including Kaposi's sarcoma.

℞ **DaunoXome®** *See* Daunorubicin Citrate Liposome Injection.

**DCIS** *See* Ductal Carcinoma In Situ.

**debulk** *See* Cytoreductive Surgery.

℞ **Decadron®** *See* Dexamethasone.

℞ **Declomycin®** *See* Demeclocycline Hydrochloride.

℞ **Deltasone®** *See* Prednisone.

℞ **demeclocycline hydrochloride** Also known by the trade name Declomycin®, this drug belongs to a group of antibiotics known as tetracyclines.

℞ **Demerol®** *See* Meperidine Hydrochloide.

℞ **denileukin diftitox** Also known by the trade name Ontak®, this is a new agent known as a fusion protein. This drug is composed of interleukin-2 (IL-2) fused to diphtheria toxin. It attaches to specific cancer cells with receptors for IL-2 and is used to treat recurrent cutaneous cell lymphoma.

**Denver® shunt** A device to remove malignant ascites (abdominal fluid caused by cancer). It consists of two plastic tubes connected by a one-way valve. Under local anesthesia, the larger tube is positioned in the abdomen, and the smaller one is placed in the large jugular vein in the neck. By pressing on the valve under the skin fluid is pumped into venous blood, carried to the kidneys, and removed in urine. Unlike paracentesis (needle drainage) that discards protein-rich ascitic fluid, a shunt removes only excess water and minerals. *See also* Ascites; LeVeen Shunt; Paracentesis; Shunt.

℞ **deodorized tincture of opium** Also known by the trade names DTO® and Laudanum®, this drug is an opioid antidiarrheal agent.

**DES** *See* Diethylstilbestrol.

**descending colon** The third section of the colon that continues downward on the left side of the abdomen. *See also* Colon.

℞ **desipramine hydrochloride** Also known by the trade names Norpramin® and Pertofrane®, this drug belongs to a group of drugs known as tricyclic antidepressants.

℞ **Desyrel®** *See* Trazodone Hydrochloride.

℞ **dexamethasone** Also known by the trade name Decadron®, this potent synthetic hormone, similar to cortisol and hydrocortisone, is used to reduce brain swelling due to tumors. It is also used to treat leukemias, lymphomas, myeloma, and Hodgkin's disease. Among the adverse effects are increased stomach acid, elevated blood glucose (sugar) level, fluid retention, and decreased resistance to infections such as tuberculosis.

℞ **dexrazoxane** Also known by the trade name Zinecard®, this drug belongs to a group of drugs known as cardioprotective agents, which protect the heart from damage. It may be used by people who are being treated with chemotherapeutic drugs, such as Adriamycin®, which can cause damage to the heart muscle.

**DHT** *See* Dihydrotestosterone.

**diabetes mellitus** A chronic metabolic disease with elevated blood sugar (blood glucose) from either a lack of insulin (Type 1 diabetes) or from a deficiency or defect of insulin utilization by cells in the body (Type 2 diabetes). It is found in all ages, and over the last decade has increased over 40% in incidence in the United States. Diabetes is associated with an increased risk for cancer of the pancreas, liver (hepatocellular or hepatoma), kidney, and uterus (endometrium).

**diaphanography** A method of examining the breast used primarily in women less than 40 years old. The technique uses bright light to illuminate inner structures. This method has limitations and, by itself, is not an adequate method of examination. *See* Appendix for Cancer Detection Guidelines.

**diaphragm** The thin muscular structure that separates the chest and abdomen; the upper surface is covered with pleura lining the chest and the under surface is covered by peritoneum enveloping the abdomen. In Hodgkin's disease, the extent or stage of the disease is derived from the involvement of lymph nodes above or below the diaphragm.

℞ **diazepam** Also known by the trade name Valium®, this is an anxiety reliever that belongs to a group of drugs known as benzodiazepines.

℞ **dicloxacillin sodium** Also known by the trade names Dycill®, Dynapen®, and Pathocil®, this drug is an antibiotic that belongs to a group of drugs known as penicillins.

℞ **Didronel®** *See* Etidronate Disodium.

**dietary fat** Although diets high in animal fats have been associated with cancer of the colon, breast, and prostate in the United States, the correlation is not strong. For breast cancer, the relation may result from obesity stemming from a high-fat intake, rather than the dietary fat itself.

℞ **diethylstilbestrol** Also known as DES, this is a synthetic female hormone associated with vaginal and cervical cancers in young girls whose mothers took the drug to prevent miscarriage. Daughters of women who received DES during pregnancy should be monitored closely and have regular pelvic examinations after their first menstrual period. Although this hormone is occasionally used in men to treat prostate cancer, it is no longer given to women of childbearing age.

**differentiation** Resemblance of a cancer to the normal tissue or the organ in which it arises as determined by microscopic examination. Tumor differentiation is used to predict the probable growth of cancer and determine treatment.

*Grade I:* Well differentiated cancer that resembles the normal tissue or organ in which it arises.

*Grade II:* Moderately differentiated cancer that slightly resembles the site of origin.

*Grade III:* Poorly differentiated or undifferentiated cancer that does not resemble any normal tissue or organ.

As a rule, well-differentiated cancers grow more slowly and spread later than do less differentiated ones. Poorly differentiated cancers may require more aggressive treatment because of the their tendency to recur following treatment.

℞ **Diflucan®** *See* Fluconazole.

**digestive tract** The long tube-like passage from mouth to anus that includes the esophagus, stomach, small and large intestine through which food is digested, water is absorbed, and solid waste is stored and eliminated. Also called alimentary canal; gastrointestinal (GI) tract.

**digital mammography** A method of storing an x-ray image of the breast as a computer image rather than on the usual x-ray film. Digital mammography can be combined with computer-assisted diagnosis, a process in which the radiologist uses the computer to help interpret the mammogram. *See also* Mammogram.

**digital rectal exam (DRE)** A physical examination used for the early detection of cancer. The doctor inserts a gloved finger into the rectum to feel for anything not normal. Some tumors of the rectum and prostate gland can be felt during a DRE. *See* Appendix for Cancer Detection Guidelines.

**dihydrotestosterone (DHT)** A powerful form of the male hormone produced by the action of a prostate enzyme on testosterone.

℞ **Dilaudid®** *See* Hydromorphone.

**dimpling** A pucker or indentation of the skin; on the breast, it may be a sign of cancer. *See also* Breast Cancer (pages 159–161).

℞ **diphenhydramine hydrochloride** Also known by the trade name Benadryl®, this drug belongs to a general group of drugs known as antihistamines. Most commonly used to treat allergies and symptoms of upper respiratory infections, it is also used to treat nausea and vomiting caused by chemotherapy.

℞ **diphenoxylate hydrochloride and atropine** Also known by the trade name Lomotil®, this drug combination is an antidiarrheal agent.

℞ **Disalcid®** *See* Salsalate.

**dissection** Surgery used to divide, separate, or remove tissues.

**diuresis** Purposely enhanced production of watery, dilute urine either by increased fluid intake or diuretic drugs (mannitol). Used to protect the kidney from the effects of cisplatin and the bladder from the effects of cyclophosphamide.

℞ **diuretic** Any drug that causes diuresis. Two of the most widely used diuretics are furosemide, given by mouth or intravenously, and mannitol, given intravenously. *See also* Furosemide; Mannitol.

**DNA** Deoxyribonucleic acid is the material that makes up genes, the basic units of heredity present in chromosomes at the nucleus (center) of every cell. It is responsible for the growth and characteristics of animals, plants, bacteria, and some viruses. *See also* Chromosome.

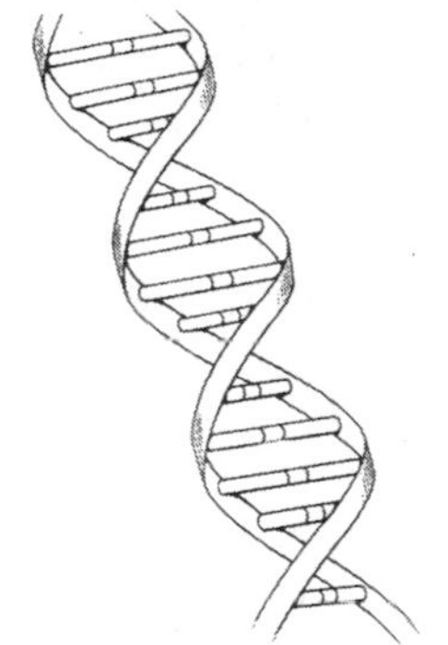

ladder shape of DNA molecules

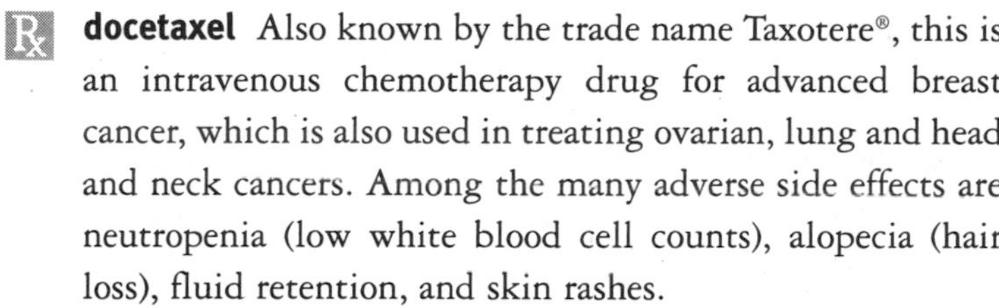

**docetaxel** Also known by the trade name Taxotere®, this is an intravenous chemotherapy drug for advanced breast cancer, which is also used in treating ovarian, lung and head and neck cancers. Among the many adverse side effects are neutropenia (low white blood cell counts), alopecia (hair loss), fluid retention, and skin rashes.

**docusate calcium, docusate potassium, docusate sodium** Also known by a number of trade names, such as Colace®, these drugs belong to a class of drugs known as stool softeners. They are used to treat constipation.

**dolasetron mesylate** Also known by the trade name Anzemet®, this drug (given intravenously) is used for treating nausea and vomiting associated with cancer chemotherapy.

**Dolophine®** *See* Methadone.

**double contrast barium enema** *See* Barium Enema.

**doubling time** The time it takes for a cell to divide and double itself. Cancer cells vary in doubling times from 8 to 600 days, averaging 100 to 120 days. Thus, a cancer may be present for many years before it can become large enough to be detected.

**doxepin hydrochloride** Also known by the trade name Sinequan®, this drug is an antidepressant related to tricyclic antidepressants.

**Doxil®** *See* Doxorubicin Hydrochloride Liposome Injection.

**doxorubicin** Also known by the trade name Adriamycin®, this antitumor antibiotic is used as chemotherapy for a variety of malignancies, which include breast, lung, prostate, and ovarian cancers; acute leukemias; Hodgkin's disease and other lymphomas; and sarcomas. The most noticeable adverse effect is temporary loss of hair, but the most serious side effect is cardiomyopathy (injury to the heart), which occurs with higher doses. Because it can injure skin and other tissue, care must be taken to prevent it from leaking from the vein when giving the drug intravenously.

℞ **doxorubicin hydrochloride liposome injection** Also known by the trade name Doxil®, this drug belongs to a group of drugs known as anthracycline antibiotics that are lipid encapsulated. It is used to treat several types of cancer, including Kaposi's sarcoma.

℞ **dronabinol** Also known by the trade name Marinol®, this drug belongs to a group of drugs known as cannabinoids, which are derived from marijuana. It is used to treat nausea and vomiting associated with chemotherapy.

℞ **droperidol** Also known by the trade name Inapsine®, this drug belongs to a group of drugs known as butyrophenones. It is used to treat nausea and vomiting following chemotherapy.

**drug resistance** The ability of a cancer cell to become resistant to the effects of chemotherapy drugs used to treat the cancer.

℞ **DTIC-Dome®** *See* Dacarbazine.

℞ **DTO®** *See* Deodorized Tincture of Opium.

**duct ectasia** A widening of the ducts of the breast, often related to breast inflammation called periductal mastitis. Duct ectasia is a condition. Symptoms are a nipple discharge, swelling, retraction of the nipple, or a lump that can be felt.

**ductal carcinoma in situ (DCIS)** The earliest stage of breast cancer; limited to the tube-like ducts that carry milk from milk-forming glands to the nipple. It is classified as either comedo or non-comedo and is similar to other in situ cancers (skin, cervical). DCIS does not metastasize (spread) to lymph nodes or other organs until it becomes invasive (grows deeper to involve breast tissue surrounding the ducts). Today, DCIS is diagnosed most often by mammograms in which it appears as a cluster of small, calcified particles. The ideal treatment for this very early-stage breast cancer is uncertain. Lumpectomy (removal of the lesion together with a rim of surrounding tissue) is the usual treatment and may include one or two lymph nodes under the arm for biopsy. *See also* Breast Cancer (pages 159–161); Mammogram.

**Dukes' classification** The first practical system to identify the extent (stage) of colorectal cancer. Derived from depth of cancer penetration into bowel wall and the presence or absence of metastasis (spread) to adjacent lymph (regional) node(s) or other parts of the body. This uncomplicated system assigns cancer of the colon and rectum to one of four stages. Stage A: cancer confined to bowel wall; Stage B: cancer penetrating through bowel wall; Stage C: cancer spread to adjacent lymph node(s); and stage D: cancer spread to other organs in the body, such as the lungs or liver. Although more precise staging methods based upon the Dukes' system (Kirkland, TNM, Astler-Coller, AJCC) have largely replaced the original method, the term "Dukes' level" is still commonly used to describe the extent of colon and rectal cancers. *See also* Colorectal Cancer (pages 163–165).

℞ **Dulcolax®** *See* Bisacodyl.

**duodenum** The upper 10 inches or so of small intestine that extends from the stomach to the jejunum (mid small intestine) into which the common bile duct and pancreatic ducts drain bile and pancreatic juice. It is often the site of benign peptic ulcer, but it is rarely the site of cancer. *See also* Intestine; Small Intestine Cancer (pages 201–202).

℞ **Duraclon®** *See* Clonidine Hydrochloride.

℞ **Duramorph®** *See* Morphine.

℞ **Dycill®** *See* Dicloxacillin Sodium.

℞ **Dynacin®** *See* Minocycline Hydrochloride.

℞ **Dynapen®** *See* Dicloxacillin Sodium.

**dysphagia** Difficulty in swallowing, often first noted while eating bread or meat, which may vary from slight chest discomfort to food sticking in the throat; usually the first symptom of esophageal cancer. Even the most minimal swallowing problem should prompt immediate attention and evaluation either by barium swallow or esophagoscopy. *See also* Barium Swallow; Esophageal Cancer (pages 167–168); Esophagoscopy.

**dysplasia** A term used by pathologists to describe abnormal cells obtained by Pap test or other biopsies. In many cases, dysplasia is the first step in the progression of normal tissue to cancers of the cervix, oral cavity, and bladder. *See also* Pap Test.

**dysplastic nevus** An abnormal mole most often on the chest, back, and abdomen, which is usually flat, larger than the end of a pencil eraser, and multicolored with an irregular border. People with dysplastic nevi are at increased risk of developing melanoma. *See also* Dysplastic Nevus Syndrome; Melanoma (pages 182–184); Skin Cancer (pages 199–201).

**dysplastic nevus syndrome** An inherited condition in which large numbers of dysplastic nevi occur in family members of people with malignant melanoma. *See also* Dysplasic Nevus; Melanoma (pages 182–184).

# E

**eccrine cancer** Any one of a variety of rare skin cancers that involve sweat glands; usually located on the head and neck or on the arms and legs. *See also* Skin Cancer (pages 199–201).

**edema** An unnatural accumulation of watery fluid in tissue (lymphedema, cerebral edema). *See also* Cerebral Edema; Lymphedema.

℞ **Effexor®** *See* Venlafaxine Hydrochloride.

**effusion** Excess fluid surrounding the lung (pleural effusion) or heart (pericardial effusion), both of which cause increasing shortness of breath. Malignant pleural effusion is caused by cancer in the chest. Initial treatment is drainage with a needle or tube; and if fluid returns, either bleomycin or talcum powder can be put into the chest, causing the lung to stick to the inside of the chest wall and obliterating the space in which fluid collects. For recurring pericardial effusion, pericardiectomy, or removal of the pericardium (sac surrounding the heart), may be needed.

℞ **Efudex®** *See* Fluorouracil.

℞ **Elavil®** *See* Amitriptyline Hydrochloride.

℞ **Eldisine®** *See* Vindesine.

**electrofulguration** A type of treatment that destroys cancer cells by burning with an electrical current.

℞ **Ellence®** *See* Epirubicin Hydrochloride.

℞ **Elspar®** *See* Asparaginase.

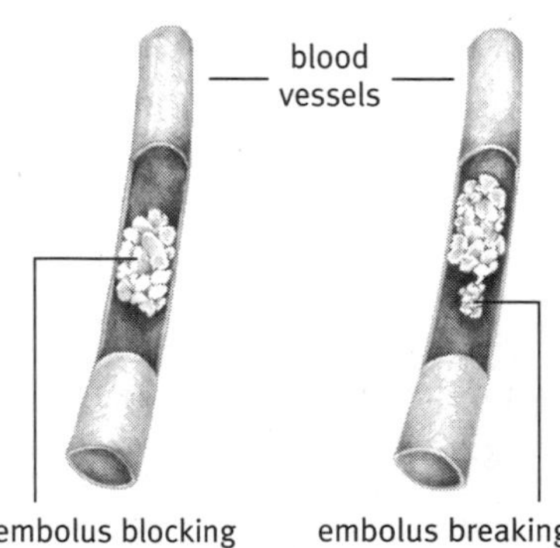


**embolism** Blockage of an artery or vein from an embolus; a fragment of a blood clot breaking free from a larger clot (thrombus) in another blood vessel. A pulmonary embolism that blocks the large artery to one or both lungs is a life-threatening emergency and is usually caused by clots in the leg and pelvic veins. It is likely to occur following operations and prolonged bed rest in people with malignant disease, especially pancreatic cancer. The anticoagulant drugs heparin or warfarin are used both to prevent and treat embolism. *See also* Heparin; Pulmonary Embolism; Warfarin.

**embolus** *See* Embolism.

**embryonal carcinoma** An uncommon cancer that affects both children and adults. It occurs in many locations and organs, including the testes or ovaries, and the mediastinum (center of the chest) in both sexes. It is derived from germ cells (embryonic cells that normally migrate only to the ovaries in females and testicles in males, where they develop into sex cells that give rise to ova [eggs] or sperm).

**Emcyt®** *See* Estramustine.

**emesis** The medical term for vomiting.

**endocrine** Having to do with hormone(s), such as endocrine gland or endocrine therapy.

**endocrine gland** A gland that produces and releases very small amounts of hormones directly into the bloodstream. Among the many endocrine glands and the hormones they produce are: ovary (estrogen), testis (testosterone), pancreas (insulin), adrenal cortex (cortisol), adrenal medulla (epinephrine), and thyroid (thyroxin).

**endocrine therapy** *See* Hormone Therapy.

**Endodan®** *See* Oxycodone.

**endometrial** Relating to the endometrium. *See* Endometrial Cancer (pages 165–167).

**endometrium** The lining of the womb or uterus where an egg fertilized in either fallopian tube attaches and develops into an embryo. *See* Endometrial Cancer (pages 165–167).

**endoscope** A lighted, magnifying instrument used to examine the interior of an organ or body space, such as a laporoscope (abdomen), gastroscope (stomach), cystoscope (bladder), colonoscope (colon-rectum).

**endoscopy** A procedure using an endoscope introduced through a body opening to visualize and biopsy the interior of organs such as the stomach, bladder, and colon. Done through small incisions, this procedure enables operations to be done in the abdomen, chest, and joints, without the need for large surgical incisions.

**endothelium** The flattened layer of cells that line arteries, veins, lymph channels, and the heart. It is rarely the site of tumors (malignant or benign).

**enterostomy** A surgical opening through the skin into the gastrointestinal (GI) tract, such as an opening in the stomach (gastrostomy), jejunum (jejunostomy), or colon (colostomy).

**enucleate** To surgically shell out without breaking or cutting into (removal of a tumor from its capsule or removal of a structure such as the eye from its socket).

**enzyme** A protein substance that causes chemical changes in food and other substances without itself undergoing change. Often identified by the suffix "ase", such as amylase (starch) or lipase (fat). Digestive enzymes from the mouth, liver, pancreas, and stomach break down fat, carbohydrate, and protein into smaller, less complex molecules that are absorbed by the small intestine for energy, body repair, and growth. Enzymes can also be found inside cells.

**ependymoma** An uncommon brain or spinal cord tumor; a type of glioma that affects both children and adults. It arises in the ependyma, the thin layer of tissue or membrane lining the center of the spinal cord and ventricles of the brain that produces spinal (cerebrospinal) fluid, which surrounds the brain and spinal cord.

**epidemiology** The study of disease in populations by collecting and analyzing statistical data. In the field of cancer, epidemiologists look at how many people have cancer, who gets specific types of cancer, and what factors play a part in the development of cancer. *See also* Etiology.

**epinephrine** A potent hormone from the center of the adrenal gland (adrenal medulla), which has many effects that include raising blood pressure, increasing heart rate, and elevating blood glucose (sugar) levels. Excess epinephrine is produced by pheochromocytoma, an adrenal tumor that can be either malignant or benign (noncancerous). Also called adrenaline. *See also* Adrenaline; Norepinephrine.

℞ **epirubicin hydrochloride** Also known by the trade names Ellence® and Pharmorubicin®, it belongs to the general group of drugs known as anthracycline antibiotics. It disrupts the growth of cancer cells, and is used with other drugs to treat breast cancer after surgery and to prevent breast cancer cells from returning.

**epithelial** Relating to epithelium. *See* Epithelium

**epithelial carcinoma** Cancer arising in the epithelium of the ovary; the most common ovarian malignancy. These tumors vary from those of low malignant potential with a very excellent prognosis after treatment (borderline cancer), to those with a tendency to early spread and frequent recurrence following therapy.

**epithelium** Any thin layer of cells that make up tissues that act variously to cover the body (skin), line internal organs (mucosa), and produce hormones (glands). Epithelial tissues give rise to carcinoma, the most common adult malignancy of the respiratory, digestive, and reproductive systems, and breast.

℞ **epoetin** Also known by the trade name Procrit®, this drug is used to treat prolonged anemia in patients with cancers (other than leukemia and lymphoma) due to the effects of chemotherapy. Epoetin is a hormone produced by the kidneys, which stimulates red blood cell production by the bone marrow when given by injection (either IV or beneath the skin). The main adverse effect is increased blood pressure.

**Epstein-Barr virus** The known cause of infectious mononucleosis, an easily spread (contagious) disease of young people. It may be responsible for several different cancers, including Hodgkin's disease, lymphoma, and throat cancer. *See also* Infectious Mononucleosis.

℞ **Ergamisol®** *See* Levamisole.

℞ **Erythrocin®** *See* Erythromycin.

**erythrocyte** *See* Red Blood Cell (RBC).

℞ **erythromycin** Also known by the trade names Ilotycin® and Erythrocin®, this is an antibiotic belonging to the macrolide class of antibiotics. It is used to treat common infections of the upper and lower respiratory tracts and sinuses. It can be used in patients who have penicillin allergies.

**esophageal** Relating to the esophagus. *See* Esophageal Cancer (pages 167–168).

**esophageal speech** An artificial method to restore the voice; used after total laryngectomy that removes the larynx (voice box). Swallowed air burped and formed by the lips provides easily understood speech without the need for a vibrating device pressed against the neck. *See* Tracheoesophageal Puncture.

**esophagectomy** Surgical removal of the esophagus. *See also* Esophageal Cancer (pages 167–168).

**esophagoscope** A lighted, usually flexible, magnifying instrument to examine and biopsy the esophagus.

**esophagoscopy** A procedure that uses an esophagoscope passed down the throat, which can be done on an outpatient basis under local and anesthesia and sedation. *See also* Esophageal Cancer (pages 167–168).

**esophagus** Part of the digestive system lined with squamous and glandular epithelium, about 10 inches long, between the pharynx (throat) and stomach. It is made up of three parts: the cervical region in the neck, the thoracic region in the chest, and the abdominal region below the diaphragm. *See also* Esophageal Cancer (pages 167–168).

℞ **Estracyt®** *See* Estramustine.

℞ **estramustine** Also known by the trade names Estracyt® and Emcyt®, this drug is a combination of an alkylating agent (nitrogen mustard) and an estrogen (estradiol phosphate). It is primarily used in the treatment of metastatic prostate cancer.

**estrogen** A general term for the female hormone produced mainly in the ovaries that is responsible for feminine traits such as body contour, head and pubic hair pattern, breast and genital development, and child bearing. Because the level of estrogen in blood markedly decreases at menopause, replacement hormone by tablet or skin patch is often used to reduce hot flashes, help prevent osteoporosis (thinning of bone), and decrease the risk of heart attack. Because replacement estrogen may slightly increase the risk of developing breast cancer, most women with a history of this malignancy are usually advised not to take the hormone, at least until they have been free of cancer for many years and are likely cured. Today, estrogen is no longer used to treat advanced prostate cancer, having been replaced by medication such as leuprolide and flutamide, both of which are less likely to lead to heart attack.

**estrogen receptor** The molecular site within breast, uterus, and other cells influenced by estrogen to which the hormone binds (attaches) and controls cellular growth and development. Breast cancers containing estrogen receptors (ER+) respond to hormone manipulation, either with tamoxifen (Nolvadex®) and other hormonal therapy drugs, or oophorectomy (removal of the ovaries), and usually are less aggressive than are cancers that lack estrogen receptors (ER-) and fail to respond to hormone treatment.

℞ **Ethyol®** *See* Amifostine.

℞ **etidronate disodium** Also known by the trade name Didronel®, this drug belongs to a group of drugs known as biphosphonates. It is a calcium-lowering drug, and is used to prevent bone from breaking down.

**etiology** The cause of a disease. In cancer, there are many probable causes, although research is showing that both genetics and life styles are major factors in many cancers. *See also* Epidemiology.

℞ **etoposide** Also known as VP-16 and by the trade name VePesid®, this chemotherapy drug is given intravenously or orally to treat testicular, lung, and bladder cancers, as well as Kaposi's sarcoma and choriocarcinoma. Adverse effects include decreased numbers of white blood cells from the toxic effect on bone marrow, mild hair loss, nausea, and vomiting.

℞ **Eulexin®** *See* Flutamide.

**EUS** Endoscopic ultrasonography uses sound waves to provide images or sonograms of the esophagus and rectum, which indicate depth of cancer penetration and presence of enlarged adjacent lymph nodes assumed to contain tumor. The probe that generates and captures sound waves is contained in the esophagoscope or colonoscope. Although not widely available, EUS appears to be the most accurate method for preoperatively staging or determining the extent of both esophageal and rectal cancers.

**Ewing's sarcoma** A cancer of bone that involves adjacent tissue, most often seen in the thighs of adolescent boys. In addition to painful swelling, this variety of bone cancer may cause generalized symptoms including fever and poor feeling, as well as increased numbers of white blood cells. Although the cancer is very responsive to radiation therapy, surgical removal and chemotherapy may improve results of treatment. *See also* Bone Cancer (pages 156–157).

**examinations for cancer** *See* Appendix.

**excisional biopsy** A surgical procedure to remove an entire growth for inspection and microscopic examination. For small cancers of the skin, excisional biopsy provides all the treatment needed. *See also* Biopsy.

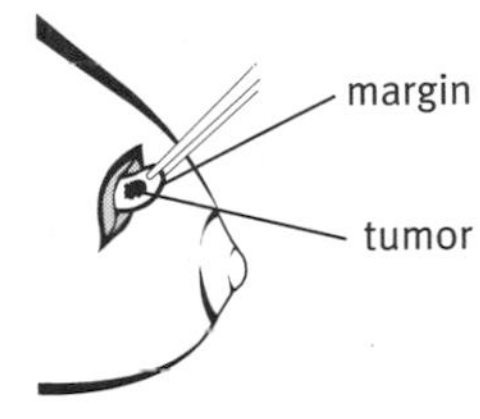

excisional biopsy

℞ **exemestane** Also known by the trade name Aromasin®, it belongs to a general group of drugs known as hormone antagonists. This drug selectively prevents the adrenal glands and ovaries from making estrogen. It is used for the treatment of advanced breast cancer in postmenopausal women whose cancer has progressed with tamoxifen therapy.

**external beam radiation** A procedure in which radiation is focused from a source outside the body on an area affected by cancer. Also called teletherapy. *See also* Radiation Therapy.

**eye cancer** *See* Retinoblastoma (pages 196–197); Uveal Melanoma.

# F

**fallopian tube** One of a pair of structures, each adjacent to the upper part of the uterus, in which an egg from the ovary is fertilized and passed into the uterus, or womb, where it develops as an embryo and later as a fetus. Tubal cancer is a rare malignancy with symptoms and treatment similar to ovarian cancer.

**false negative** A test result implying that a condition does not exist when in fact it does.

**false positive** A test result implying that a condition exists when in fact it does not.

℞ **famciclovir** Also known by the trade name Famvir®, this drug belongs to a group of drugs known as antiviral agents. It is used to treat a variety of herpesviruses.

**familial adenomatous polyposis** An inherited precancerous condition of the colon and rectum with adenomatous polyps (small mushroom-like growths) present in the mucosa (lining). Polyps can also occur in other portions of the gastrointestinal tract as well. It usually becomes evident in late childhood when rectal bleeding occurs. Cancer will almost invariably develop unless the involved intestine is removed before the polyps undergo malignant change. In cases where the lower rectum is not removed, colonoscopy is repeated every 6 months to destroy newly formed polyps with electrocautery (electric current). The drug celecoxib, most commonly used to treat arthritis, is used to reduce the number of polyps in individuals with this disease. *See also* Colorectal Cancer (pages 163–165).

**familial cancer syndrome** *See* Cancer Family Syndrome.

℞ **Famvir®** *See* Famciclovir.

℞ **Fareston®** *See* Toremifene.

**fat necrosis** The death of fat cells, usually following injury. Fat necrosis is a benign condition, but it can cause a breast lump, pulling of the skin, or skin changes that can be confused with breast cancer.

**fatigue** The feeling of decreased mental and physical activity often accompanied by sleepiness or irritability; the most common side effect of cancer chemotherapy. This problem, which is often unrecognized and not adequately treated, is frequently due to anemia that results from the harmful effects of anticancer drugs on bone marrow.

**fecal occult blood test** A simple, inexpensive test to reveal occult (unrecognized) blood in a stool sample, which can indicate cancer of the intestinal tract, especially of the colon and rectum. It is advised as part of the yearly physical examination in men and women 50 years of age and older, unless there is a family history of colon cancer or other indication of high risk. *See* Appendix for Cancer Detection Guidelines; Colorectal Cancer (pages 163–165).

℞ **Femara®** *See* Letrozole.

℞ **fentanyl citrate** Also known by the trade name Actiq®, this is an opioid used to relieve moderate to severe breakthrough pain.

℞ **fentanyl transdermal system** Also known by the trade name Duragesic®, this is a potent opioid, often applied as a skin patch.

**fever** A body temperature greater than 98.6°F, which in a cancer patient may be the first and only indication of infection. Anyone receiving chemotherapy who has a white blood cell count of less than 500 granulocytes or neutrophils (normal = 3,500–10,500) is at increased risk for serious bacterial infection. Any individual who develops either an oral temperature of 100.4°F on three occasions taken 4 hours apart or a temperature of 101°F (on one occasion) should immediately contact a physician.

℞ **Fiberall®** *See* Psyllium Hydrophobic Muciloid.

**fibroadenoma** A common, benign (noncancerous) breast tumor of young women, which is usually firm, round, non-tender, and moveable. Rarely do these benign growths become very large and develop into cancer.

**fibrocystic changes (disease)** A benign (noncancerous) condition of the female breast, which causes fluid-filled cysts and firm areas that are often confused with cancer. This condition occurs most often in middle-aged and younger women, but may occur in older women receiving estrogen. A form of fibrocystic disease, atypical hyperplasia is associated with an increased risk of breast cancer, particularly in women with a family history of breast malignancy.

**fibrolamellar carcinoma** An uncommon variety of cancer that originates in the liver (primary liver cancer or hepatoma), which is slower growing and more responsive to surgical removal than the usual hepatocellular carcinoma. This type of liver malignancy does not usually produce alpha fetoprotein, used as tumor marker in most cases of hepatoma. *See also* Liver Cancer (pages 178–179).

**fibrosarcoma** A type of soft tissue (nonbone) cancer that arises in fibrous tissue (tissue that connects structures and organs in the body). This form of sarcoma occurs at any age, but is most commonly seen in people 30 to 55 years of age. *See also* Sarcoma; Soft Tissue Cancer (pages 202–204).

**fibrosis** The formation of fibrous, scar-like tissue that can occur anywhere in the body.

℞ **filgrastim** Also known by the trade name Neupogen®, this is a cytokine that belongs to a class of artificially synthesized drugs known as biological response modifiers. It is used to increase the number of infection-fighting white blood cells after chemotherapy.

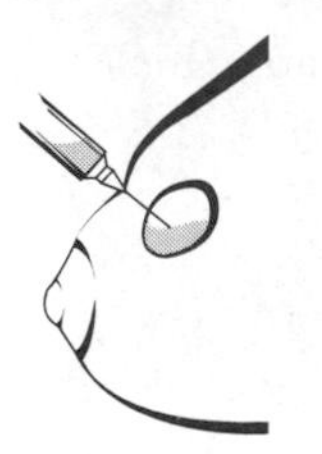
fine needle aspiration biopsy

**fine needle aspiration (FNA)** A biopsy to examine fluid or small pieces of tissue drawn up through a small needle, which is safe, simple, and virtually painless. FNA is often used to evaluate lumps in breast and thyroid, and sample enlarged lymph nodes. Using x-ray or ultrasound guidance, the technique is used to biopsy tumors inside the chest and abdomen. *See also* Biopsy.

**first-degree relative** A parent, sibling, or child of a person.

**fistula** An abnormal passage or communication between two internal organs, or an internal organ and skin. It is often caused by advanced-stage cancers invading surrounding tissue.

**five-year survival rate** The percentage of people with a given cancer who are expected to survive 5 years or longer with a disease. Five-year survival rates are used to produce a standard way of discussing prognosis. *See also* Survival Rate.

℞ **Flagyl®** *See* Metronidazole Hydrochloride.

**flare** A temporary increase in bone pain or tumor size experienced by 10% to 15% of women with advanced-stage breast cancer who begin hormone therapy with tamoxifen (Nolvadex®). It occurs shortly after the drug is started and usually lasts only a short time. Surprisingly, it often indicates an ultimately good response to treatment with tamoxifen.

**flexible sigmoidoscopy** *See* Sigmoidoscopy.

**flow cytometry** A laboratory procedure using a laser technique to analyze individual cells for DNA content, estimate their number of chromosomes (ploidy), and the fraction of cells replicating their DNA (S-phase fraction, which reflects the rate at which a cell is reproducing). The technique is used to distinguish benign (noncancerous) lymphatic conditions from malignancies (lymphoma, leukemia), identify subtypes of cancer, and predict growth rate and possible outcome of some cancers.

℞ **floxuridine** Also known by the trade name FUDR®, this is an antimetabolite chemotherapy drug similar to fluorouracil (5-FU). It is given by artery to treat head and neck cancer, and cancer spread into the liver. When administered by the hepatic artery to the liver, FUDR® can produce cholangitis (severe irritation of the common duct) that causes the duct to narrow and block the flow of bile from the liver, which results in jaundice.

℞ **fluconazole** Also known by the trade name Diflucan®, this drug is belongs to the azole group of drugs. It is use to treat fungal infections.

℞ **flucytosine** Also known by the trade name Ancobon®, this drug is an antifungal agent.

℞ **Fludara®** *See* Fludarabine Phosphate.

℞ **fludarabine phosphate** Also known by the trade name Fludara®, this drug belongs to a group of drugs known as antimetabolites. It is used to treat some types of leukemia, including chronic lymphocytic leukemia.

℞ **fluorouracil** Also known as 5-FU, this is an antimetabolite-type of chemotherapy drug, usually given intravenously to treat a variety of cancers, including breast, colorectal, and liver. Efudex® skin cream and liquid containing this drug are used for small basal cell skin cancers as well as for keratoses (benign skin growths). The adverse side effects of the intravenous administration of this drug include bone marrow toxicity, mouth irritation, diarrhea, and hair loss.

℞ **fluoxetine hydrochloride** Also known by the trade name Prozac®, this drug belongs to a group of drugs known as antidepressants.

℞ **flusol DA (20%)** This investigational drug belongs to a group of drugs known as radiosensitizers, which enhance the effectiveness of radiation on cancer cells.

℞ **flutamide** Also known by the trade name Eulexin®, this is an oral, antiandrogen drug that blocks the effects of the male hormone (androgen) on the prostate; used to treat advanced prostate cancer. It is usually given together with a leuteinizing hormone-releasing hormone (LHRH), such as leuprolide, that causes a medical castration, the effects of which are similar to orchiectomy (removal of the testicles).

**FNA** *See* Fine Needle Aspiration.

℞ **Folex®** *See* Methotrexate.

**folinic acid** *See* Leucovorin.

**follicular adenoma** A benign (noncancerous) thyroid tumor that may be mistaken, especially in a needle biopsy, for follicular thyroid cancer. *See* Follicular Carcinoma.

**follicular carcinoma** A variety of thyroid cancer that accounts for approximately 10% of all malignant thyroid tumors, often difficult to distinguish from follicular adenoma (a benign tumor of the thyroid). Follicular carcinoma tends to spread through blood rather than via lymph nodes, as does the more common papillary thyroid cancer. *See also* Thyroid Cancer (pages 207–209).

**follicular lymphoma** A type of adult lymphoma, which primarily affects lymph nodes, bone marrow, and spleen. Although it is usually not curable, it is generally a slow growing malignancy. *See also* Non-Hodgkin's Lymphoma (pages 188–190).

℞ **Fortaz®** *See* Ceftazidime.

℞ **foscarnet sodium** Also known by the trade name Foscavir®, this drug belongs to a group of drugs known as antiviral agents. It is used to treat infections with herpesviruses that do not respond to other treatments, and viral eye infections.

℞ **Foscavir®** *See* Foscarnet Sodium.

**fracture** Any break, especially involving bone. A pathologic fracture is one that occurs in diseased bone, either from bone cancer originating in the skeleton, or cancer spread from another site, such as breast or prostate.

**free-PSA ratio** A ratio that indicates how much prostate-specific antigen (PSA) circulates alone, or unbound, in the blood, and how much is bound together with other blood proteins. A low percent free PSA (25% or less) suggests that prostate cancer is more likely to be present and suggests the need for a biopsy. *See also* Prostate-Specific Antigen.

**frozen section** A laboratory technique that enables tissue samples to be processed quickly for analysis under the microscope; invaluable in diagnosing and staging malignant disease. Biopsy specimens are quickly frozen and cut into very thin slices (sections) for staining and viewing. Although the details in frozen sections are not as precise as those obtained in permanent sections that require at least 12 hours for processing, they usually enable the pathologist to distinguish cancer from benign tissue. The technique is not applicable to bone biopsies that require decalcifying, a softening process taking several days.

℞ **FUDR®** *See* Floxuridine.

℞ **Fungizone®** *See* Amphotericin B (Amphotericin B Lipid Complex).

**fungus** A broad variety of primitive organisms, including molds and yeasts; originally the source of antibacterial antibiotics (penicillin, streptomycin) and anticancer antibiotics (doxorubicin, bleomycin). Although they rarely cause problems in healthy individuals, fungi can produce severe infections in people with weakened immune systems from conditions such as AIDS. People receiving multiple antibacterial antibiotics for long periods are prone to develop fungal infection in the mouth (thrush) and vagina.

℞ **furosemide** Also known by the trade name Lasix®, this is a diuretic drug that increases urine flow from the kidneys. It is used for removing excess fluid from the body. By diluting the urine, it can help prevent kidney injury in cancer patients receiving cisplatin, and bladder injury (cystitis) in those receiving cyclophosphamide. *See also* Diuretic; Mannitol.

# G

℞ **gabapentin** Also known by the trade name Neurontin®, this drug belongs to a group of drugs known as anticonvulsants. It is used in the treatment of neuropathic pain.

**gallbladder** *See* Gallbladder Cancer (pages 168–170).

℞ **gallium nitrate** Also known by the trade name Ganite®, this drug belongs to a group of drugs known as hypocalcemic agents. It is used to prevent bone from breaking down (calcium loss) and to treat elevated calcium levels in patients with cancer.

**gamma knife** *See* Stereotactic Radiosurgery.

**gamma ray** A beam of high-energy x-rays from both natural and artificially-made radioactive isotopes (radionuclides) used to diagnose cancer by means of a sensing device or scanner passed over the body; also used to treat malignant tumors. Radioactive scans identify cancers of bone, liver, and thyroid, and more recently, sentinel node(s) in melanoma and breast cancer.

℞ **ganciclovir** Also known by the trade name Cytovene®, this drug belongs to a group of drugs known as antiviral agents. It is used to treat infections with herpesviruses, Epstein-Barr virus, and cytomegalovirus.

**ganglioma** *See* Ganglioneuroma.

**ganglioneuroma** A benign (noncancerous) nerve tumor of older children and adults, most often found in the posterior mediastinum (chest) and retroperitoneum (abdomen), sometimes in relation to the adrenal gland. The very malignant childhood tumor, neuroblastoma, occasionally may mature into a ganglioneuroma. Also called ganglioma.

℞ **Ganite®** *See* Gallium Nitrate.

℞ **Garamycin®** *See* Gentamicin Sulfate.

**Gardner's syndrome** Multiple polyps that develop at a young age that have a predisposition to cancer, usually of the colon. It can also cause benign tumors of the skin, soft connective tissue, and bones.

**gastrectomy** Surgical removal or excision of the stomach, either complete (total) or partial (subtotal); the mainstay for treating stomach cancer. *See also* Stomach Cancer (pages 204–206).

**gastric** Pertaining to the stomach.

**gastrin** A hormone from the lining of lower part of the stomach (gastric antrum) that causes the stomach to produce acid.

**gastrinoma** A gastrin-producing tumor associated with the Zollinger-Ellison syndrome, which is cancerous in 60% to 90% of cases. It occurs most often in the pancreas and less commonly in the upper part of the small intestine (duodenum).

**gastritis** Inflammation of the stomach; a particular form of gastritis called atrophic gastritis results in decreased absorption of vitamin $B_{12}$ and decreased acid in the stomach. Atrophic gastritis is associated with an increased risk of developing cancer in the stomach. *See also* Stomach Cancer (pages 204–206).

**gastroesophageal junction (GEJ)** The GEJ is where the lower end of the esophagus joins the proximal (upper) part of the stomach; increasingly the site of the adenocarcinoma variety of esophageal cancer. *See also* Esophageal Cancer (pages 167–168).

**gastrointestinal (GI)** Relating to stomach and intestines. *See also* Digestive Tract.

**gastroscope** A lighted magnifying instrument (endoscope) passed down the throat to view and biopsy the stomach.

**gastroscopy** Procedure to examine the interior of the stomach with a gastroscope, usually done under local anesthesia with sedatives.

**gastrostomy** Surgical procedure to create an opening into the stomach; often done for feeding or draining fluid from the stomach. Also, the opening or stoma itself. Today, this procedure is often done through the gastroscope under local anesthesia. *See also* Stoma.

**G-CSF** *See* Granulocyte-Colony Stimulating Factor.

**GEJ** *See* Gastroesophageal Junction.

℞ **gemcitabine** Also known by the trade name Gemzar®, this drug belongs to a group of drugs known as antimetabolites. It is used in the treatment of pancreatic cancer and is being investigated as a treatment for some lung cancers.

℞ **Gemzar®** *See* Gemcitabine.

**gene** The basic unit of heredity that determines the characteristics of each succeeding generation. Each gene is composed of the chemical compound DNA, which occupies a specific space or locus on one of the 46 chromosomes normally present in human cells.

**gene therapy** Experimental cancer treatment in which a gene inserted into a cancer cell restores more normal growth control or makes the cell more susceptible and more likely to be killed by the body's immune (protective) mechanism. It is being investigated as therapy for many cancers including brain tumors and cancers of the ovary and colon.

**genetic counseling** The process of obtaining information about the risk of inherited disorders such as cancer, including a discussion of possible treatment alternatives available to decrease the risk of developing certain cancers. *See also* Heredity.

**genital** Relating to the female or male sex organs.

**genital herpes** An infection of the herpes simplex virus that produces vesicles (small blisters) on genitals.

**genome** The total DNA in a single cell, representing all of the genetic information of the organism.

Rx **gentamicin sulfate** Also known by the trade name Garamycin®, this drug is an antibiotic that belongs to a group of drugs known as aminoglycosides.

Rx **Geocillin®** *See* Carbenicillin Indanyl Sodium.

Rx **Geopen®** *See* Carbenicillin Indanyl Sodium.

**germ cell cancer** Any one of a variety of cancers, which arise from embryonic cells (germ cells) that normally migrate to the ovaries in females and testicles in males, where they develop into sex cells that produce ova (eggs) or sperm. Theses malignancies occur at any age. Although germ cell cancers of the testis (seminoma and nonseminoma) are the most common malignant tumors of young men (aged 20 to 35 years), germ cell tumors of the ovary are unusual in women, accounting for only 2% to 3% of all ovarian cancers in American women. In both children and adults they occur in many sites along the midline, an imaginary line from the brain to the lower end of the spine in front of and parallel to the spinal column. Also called germinoma. *See also* Testicular Cancer (pages 206–207).

**germinoma** *See* Germ Cell Cancer.

**GI** *See* Gastrointestinal.

**gland** A group of cells or an organ that produces a substance (secretion or hormone) not needed by the cell or organ in which it is produced. For instance, the salivary glands in the mouth produce saliva, a secretion that moistens food and aids in digesting starches; the pancreas releases insulin that lowers blood sugar (glucose).

**Gleason score** A method of classifying prostate cancer cells. This system applies a grade ranging from 1 to 5 to a certain area of cancer cells based on how much the arrangement looks like the way normal prostate cells are arranged in the prostate gland. Because prostate cancers often have areas with different grades, a grade is assigned to each of the two areas that make up most of the cancer. The two grades are added together to give a Gleason score between 2 and 10. The higher the number, the faster the cancer is likely to grow and the more likely it is to spread beyond the prostate. *See also* Prostate Cancer (pages 194–196).

℞ **Gleevec®** *See* STI-571.

**glioblastoma multiforme** A rapidly growing, invariably fatal, brain tumor that occurs most often in adults and can usually be identified by MRI. Surgery to remove part of the tumor, followed by radiation and often chemotherapy, is used to palliate or relieve symptoms. *See also* Brain Tumor (pages 157–159).

**glioma** A malignant tumor of the brain or spinal cord, which arises from glial tissue (tissue in the central nervous system that supports nerve tissue). Gliomas can vary from a slow growing tumor to a rapidly expanding, and universally fatal glioblastoma. *See also* Brain Tumor (pages 157–159).

℞ **Glivec®** *See* STI-571.

**glomus tumor** *See* Carotid Body Tumor.

**glucagonoma** A rare, hormone-producing cancer usually derived from cells in the islands of Langerhans (islet cells) of the pancreas, which produce glucagon that acts the opposite of insulin by increasing blood glucose (sugar). Symptoms include skin rashes and weight loss, and the diagnosis is made upon finding increased levels of glucagon in blood. The tumor is usually slow growing, and incomplete surgical removal reduces symptoms in most cases. Chemotherapy is similar to that used for treating the type of tumor (gastrinoma) that produces the hormone gastrin (gastrinoma), which is associated with the Zollinger-Ellison syndrome. *See also* Pancreatic Cancer (pages 191–193).

**glucose** The sugar component of blood, the level of which is controlled by several hormones, including insulin that lowers blood sugar and glucagon that raises it. In diabetes, glucose can be present in urine.

**gold 198** The radioisotope of gold used in radiation therapy of cancer in the form of small metallic "seeds" placed in, or adjacent to, a tumor and used as a liquid injected in the abdomen.

**gonadotropin** Any hormone that stimulates the gonads (testicles in men and ovaries in women). Beta human chorionic gonadotropin (β-hCG), normally produced by fetal tissues during pregnancy, is also produced by gestational cancers (including those of testis and ovary), in which case it is used as a tumor marker.

℞ **goserelin** Also known by the trade name Zoladex®, this is an anticancer drug used as hormone therapy for advanced prostate cancer. It produces a "medical" orchiectomy by preventing the testes from producing testosterone, the most potent male hormone. It is given by injection once a month.

**grade** *See* Differentiation.

℞ **granisetron hydrochloride** Also known by the trade name Kytril®, this drug belongs to a group of drugs known as serotonin antagonists. It is used to treat nausea.

**granulocyte** A type of white blood cell (leukocyte) produced in bone marrow; part of the body's defense mechanism that protects against bacterial infection. Many drugs used in cancer treatment are toxic or poisonous to bone marrow and reduce the number of granulocytes in blood, which can result in an overwhelming and even fatal infection. In cancer patients receiving chemotherapy, leukocyte numbers are monitored by frequent complete blood counts so that the dose of medication can be adjusted to prevent granulocytopenia (low levels of granulocytes). Also called neutrophil; polymorphonuclear leukocyte.

**granulocyte-colony stimulating factor (G-CSF)** A hormone-like protein produced in minute amounts by a variety of cells, which stimulates the granulocyte variety of white blood cells. G-CSF is used to stimulate bone marrow injured by chemotherapy or radiation therapy, especially during bone marrow (stem cell) transplant. *See also* Bone Marrow.

**granulocyte macrophage-colony stimulating factor** A substance similar to granulocyte-colony stimulating factor, which not only stimulates the growth of granulocytes in bone marrow, but also stimulates monocytes, which are large cells scattered throughout the body that destroy bacteria by engulfing them. *See also* Bone Marrow.

**granulocytopenia** A decrease in the normal number of granulocytes in blood. *See also* Granulocyte.

**granulomatous colitis** *See* Crohn's Disease.

**granulosa cell tumor** A rare cancer of the ovary or testis, which can produce large amounts of the female hormone estrogen. In young girls, this results in the appearance of adult female sexual characteristics at a very early age, such as enlarged breasts and the onset of menstruation. In males, the tumor causes gynecomastia (enlarged breasts). *See also* Ovarian Cancer (pages 190–191); Testicular Cancer (pages 206–207).

**gray (Gy)** The international unit to measure the dose of ionizing radiation absorbed by the body during cancer treatment. One Gy equals 100 rad, the older unit of radiation measurement.

℞ **grepafloxacin** Also known by the trade name Raxar®, this is an antibiotic that belongs to a group of drugs known as fluoroquinolones.

**groin dissection** Surgical removal of lymph nodes (lymphadenectomy) in the groin or inguinal area; often used to treat melanoma of the leg, lower abdomen, and back. The operation is also used to treat advanced cancers of the genital and anal area. Removal of all lymph nodes in the groin (deep lympadenectomy) often results in lymphedema (swelling) of the leg. *See also* Lymphedema.

**Gy** *See* Gray.

**gynecomastia** Enlargement of the male breast, which can be caused by estrogen and less often by flutamide taken to treat prostate cancer. It can be caused by lung and other cancers that either produce estrogen directly or produce other hormones that affect estrogen metabolism.

# H

**hair loss** *See* Alopecia.

**hairy cell leukemia** A slow growing leukemia of older people, which can be well controlled, although is probably not curable. The leukemic cells present in bone marrow appear covered with fine hair-like extensions when viewed under the microscope. It can cause splenomegaly (massive enlargement of the spleen), which often results in hypersplenism, a condition with decreased numbers of white blood cells (leukopenia), platelets (thrombocytopenia), and red blood cells (anemia). Surgical removal of the spleen (splenectomy) may be needed to control repeated infections. Hairy cell leukemia often responds to immunotherapy with interferon-alpha (IFN-$\alpha$). A number of therapies can lead to compete remission of this disease. Pentostatin, an antimetabolite chemotherapy drug, may be useful in treating disease no longer controlled by interferon. *See also* Leukemia (pages 176–178).

℞ **Haldol®** *See* Haloperidol.

℞ **haloperidol** Also known by the trade name Haldol®, this drug belongs to a group of drugs known as butyrophenones. It is used in patients with cancer to treat nausea and vomiting from chemotherapy.

**hamartoma** In an organ, a benign (noncancerous) abnormal mixture of normal tissues, or the abnormal proportion of a single tissue. Hamartomas are unlikely to compress adjacent tissue (in contrast to most other tumors).

**hCG** Human chorionic gonadotropin. *See* Beta-Human Chorionic Gonadotropin.

**head of pancreas** The larger part of the pancreas, to the right of the spine; most often the site of pancreatic cancer. Jaundice (yellow staining of eyes and skin), without abdominal pain (as occurs in gallstone disease), is the usual first indication of cancer in this location due to a tumor blocking the common bile duct, thus impeding the flow of bile from the liver. *See also* Pancreas; Pancreatic Cancer (pages 191–193).

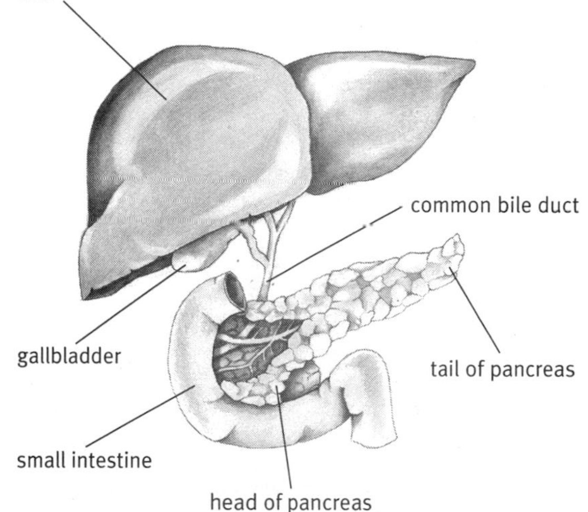


**heart disease** *See* Cardiomyopathy.

***Helicobacter pylori*** A more recently recognized variety of bacteria found to cause persistent gastritis (stomach irritation) and ulcers. Some studies suggest that infection due to *H. pylori* may cause gastric malignancies (adenocarcinoma, lymphoma) as well as Barrett's esophagus, a condition that leads to adenocarcinoma of the lower part of the esophagus. However, very few people with *Helicobacter* infection develop cancers of the stomach and esophagus.

**hematoma** A collection of blood outside a blood vessel caused by a leak or injury. Hematomas that occur in the breast after injury or surgery may feel like a lump.

**hematuria** Blood in urine, which can be severe enough to color the urine (gross hematuria) or so slight as to be recognizable only on microscopic examination (microscopic hematuria). Passing bloody urine without pain (painless hematuria) may be the first symptom of cancer of the kidney and urinary tract (ureters, bladder, urethra).

**hemipelvectomy** Surgical removal of half of the bony pelvis, along with corresponding buttock and leg, is an extensive operation to treat large cancers in the pelvic area; most often osteogenic (bone) and soft tissue sarcomas.

**hemoptysis** Coughing blood; often the first indication of lung, head, or neck cancer. Even the slightest, persistent blood-streaked sputum requires evaluation by a physician. It can also be caused by infections such as pneumonia.

℞ **heparin** This is a potent injectable drug that delays coagulation (blood clotting). It is used to prevent clots forming in arteries and veins and to treat pulmonary embolism (blood clots to the lungs). It also prevents clotting of vascular access devices. The effect of heparin is monitored either by clotting time or activated partial thromboplastin time (APTT). *See also* Clotting Time.

**hepatectomy** Partial or total surgical removal of the liver; used to treat cancer arising in the liver (primary cancer) or spread to the liver from some other sites, especially the colon and rectum. Although total hepatectomy that requires a liver transplant is used rarely to control cancer in adults, it is used to treat hepatoblastoma (liver cancer) in children. *See also* Liver Cancer (pages 178–179).

**hepatic** Relating to the liver.

**hepatitis** Inflammation of the liver, most often caused by a viral infection, but occasionally caused by alcohol abuse or exposure to chemical solvents and some medications. Hepatitis from the hepatitis B virus and the hepatitis C virus is thought to be the underlying cause of hepatoma (liver cancer), which is common in equatorial Africa. The cancer-causing effect of the viruses appears to be intensified by aflatoxin, a toxic (poisonous) substance from a fungus growing on grain and peanuts. *See also* Liver Cancer (pages 178–179).

**hepatobiliary carcinoma** *See* Liver Cancer (pages 178–179).

**hepatoblastoma** A rare, childhood liver cancer that usually affects children less than 3 years old. Swelling of the abdomen is often the first indication, and the tumor marker alpha-fetoprotein (AFP), present in blood of 75% of those affected, is used together with abdominal CT to diagnose the tumor. Although many children need only partial removal of the liver (partial hepatectomy), those with a single large or multiple tumors may require total liver resection (total hepatectomy), which makes a liver transplant necessary. In some cases, preoperative chemotherapy is used to shrink the cancer prior to surgery so that only partial removal of the liver is needed. *See also* Liver Cancer (pages 178–179).

**hepatocellular cancer** The most common variety of liver cancer that arises in the liver (primary cancer) from hepatic cells, which provide liver function and form more than 99% of the organ. Also called hepatoma. *See also* Liver Cancer (pages 178–179).

**hepatoma** *See* Hepatocellular Cancer.

**HER2/*neu*** Abnormalities (overexpression) of this gene in breast, ovary, and some other cancers are associated with tumors that grow rapidly, are more likely to metastasize (spread), and are less likely to respond to chemotherapy. Women with widespread breast cancer whose tumors test positive for this gene should be considered for treatment with Herceptin®, a drug directed toward the HER2/*neu* gene. *See also* Breast Cancer (pages 159–161); Lung Cancer (pages 180–182); Ovarian Cancer (pages 190–191); Trastuzumab.

℞ **Herceptin®** *See* Trastuzumab.

**heredity** The passing of traits from parent to offspring, such as body build, hair or eye color, etc.; increasingly recognized as having a role in the development of some cancers. Transmission between generations can occur as identifiable malignancies—retinoblastoma, medullary thyroid cancer, breast cancer, ovary cancer; premalignant conditions—multiple colon polyposis (colon cancer), dysplastic nevus (melanoma); nonmalignant conditions—Down's syndrome (childhood leukemia), Klinefelter's syndrome (male breast cancer). *See also* Inherited.

**herpesvirus** Any one of several viruses that cause a variety of infections in humans and animals. Herpes simplex causes vesicles (small blisters) on the lips or genitals, Herpes zoster causes shingles (tiny, painful blisters along the path of nerves on one side of the chest or abdomen), and the Epstein-Barr virus (EBV) causes infectious mononucleosis. EBV is thought to have a role in causing nasopharyngeal carcinoma (a type of nose and throat cancer) and some forms of lymphoma.

℞ **Hexalen®** *See* Altretamine.

℞ **Hexamethylmelamine®** *See* Altretamine.

**5-HIAA** 5-Hydroxyindoleacetic acid is a chemical compound in urine used to identify both cancerous and nonmalignant carcinoid tumors. It is produced in the kidneys from the hormone serotonin and is released in blood in excessive amounts by carcinoids. Although not always present in carcinoids, finding 5-HIAA in a urine sample collected over a 24-hour period ensures the diagnosis. Fruits (bananas, pineapple), nuts, and drugs (cough syrup) consumed or taken during the test can cause a falsely elevated level of the compound. *See also* Carcinoid.

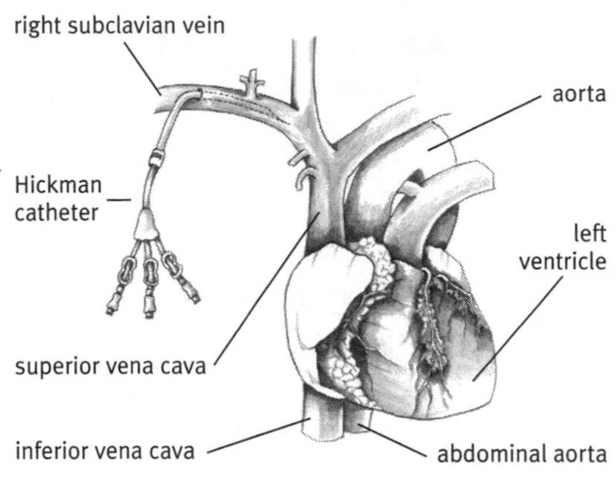


Hickman catheter.
Catheter is inserted into right subclavian vein.

**Hickman catheter** A vascular access device that consists of a small plastic tube secured in a vein and brought out through the skin; used for drawing blood and giving chemotherapy or total parental nutrition (TPN). A sponge-like plastic cuff around the tubing beneath the skin acts as a barrier to infection and anchors the device. When not in use, the catheter is capped and filled with the anticoagulant heparin to prevent blood clotting. The minor operation necessary to place the catheter can be done in outpatient surgery under local anesthesia. *See* Vascular Access Device.

**high-dose therapy** Cancer treatment with very large doses of chemotherapy and/or radiation therapy, which without bone marrow or stem cell transplant would result in severe adverse effects and probable death. This treatment is generally reserved for people who initially respond to, and later fail, more conventional cancer therapy. *See also* Chemotherapy.

**HIV** Human immunodeficiency virus that causes acquired immunodeficiency syndrome (AIDS) by weakening the body's immune (protective) mechanism. AIDS is associated with a number of different malignancies, including Kaposi's sarcoma, cervical cancer, and brain lymphoma. *See* Acquired Immunodeficiency Syndrome.

**hormonal ablation** *See* Combination Hormone Therapy.

**hormone** Any one of numerous short-lived chemical compounds produced in minute amounts by various endocrine glands which control the growth, development, and function of particular "target" organ(s) sensitive to its actions. Hormones also affect the activity of hormone-dependent cancers of breast, prostate, thyroid, and uterus. Among the most familiar hormones and their sources are insulin (pancreas), cortisol (cortisone; adrenal cortex), epinephrine (adrenal medulla), estrogen (ovary), testosterone (testis), and thyroxin (thyroid).

**hormone manipulation** *See* Hormone Therapy.

**hormone receptor** A protein molecule on the surface of cells or within cells in organs and tissues affected by hormones (breast, prostate, thyroid) that is the site to which the specific hormone attaches or binds to the cell. The presence of hormone receptors in cancer cells indicates hormone therapy is likely to be of benefit.

**hormone therapy** Treatment that alters the hormonal environment of a cancer whose growth is under hormonal control, such as breast, prostate, and thyroid cancers. Alteration can be accomplished by the following:

*Ablative therapy:* Surgical removal or medical eradication of a hormone source (removal of testes or administration of leuprolide or goserelin to eliminate the major source of the male hormone testosterone). Both surgical and medical castrations are useful in treating advanced prostate cancer.

*Additive therapy:* Medication that alters the effects of a hormone. For example, estrogen may be used to counteract testosterone in order to treat prostate cancer; tamoxifen may be used to block estrogen in order to treat breast cancer; thyroid hormone may be used to stop thyroid-stimulating hormone (TSH) in order to treat thyroid cancer. In the past, hormone therapy was used only for advanced cancers; but today, it is advised as adjuvant therapy in treating less advanced breast, uterus, and thyroid malignancies. The antiestrogen drug tamoxifen (Nolvadex®) has been found to lessen the risk of women developing breast cancer (those with atypical hyperplasia and a strong family history of breast malignancy). Also called hormone manipulation; endocrine therapy.

**Horner's syndrome** A condition with drooping eyelid (ptosis), sinking in of eye (enophthalmos), small pupil (miosis), and absence of facial sweating (mydriasis) on the side in which there is injury to a nerve (autonomic nerve) in the neck. It can be caused by lung cancer at the top of the lung (Pancoast tumor) or by trauma that sometimes occurs in the head and neck following surgery.

**hospice** An institution or organization that furnishes support for dying patients and their families. In the United States, there are approximately 2,500 hospice programs providing care to advanced cancer and other terminally ill patients and furnishing physical, psychological, spiritual, and social support services. Care is provided in the home or other setting by health care professionals and volunteers and is usually covered by insurance.

**HPC 1** Inherited DNA changes in a gene called HPC 1 may make prostate cancer more likely to develop in some men. These changes appear to be responsible for approximately 10% of prostate cancers. Research on this gene is still preliminary, and a genetic test is not yet available.

**human papillomavirus (HPV)** Any one of a large number of different viruses that cause warts on the skin of the genitals and around the anus. It is believed to be a factor in the development of most cervical cancers and in some penile, vaginal, and anal cancers. *See also* Anal Cancer (pages 152–153); Cervical Cancer (pages 161–163); Penile Cancer (pages 193–194); Vaginal Cancer (pages 209–211).

℞ **Hycamtin®** *See* Topotecan.

**hydatidiform mole** A grapelike mass in the uterus, which develops from the placenta (afterbirth) during early pregnancy. The tumor causes vaginal bleeding, and in cases in which it penetrates the uterus (chorioadenoma destruens), it causes the womb to rupture internally. It is the most common pregnancy complication that leads to choriocarcinoma, a fast growing and rapidly spreading type of gestational cancer.

℞ **Hydrea®** *See* Hydroxyurea.

℞ **hydrocortisone** *See* Cortisone.

℞ **hydromorphone** Also known by the trade name Dilaudid®, this drug is an opioid analgesic used to treat moderate to severe pain.

℞ **hydroxyurea** Also known by the trade name Hydrea®, this drug belongs to a group of drugs known as antimetabolites. It is used in the treatment of several types of cancer; it is used primarily in the treatment of chronic myelogenous leukemia.

**hyperalimentation** Giving nutrition other than solid food, often intravenously.

**hypercalcemia** An increased calcium level in the blood is a common, potentially life-threatening disorder often associated with cancer; due either to malignant tumor involving bone or to unknown substances produced by a cancer, which causes the skeleton to release calcium. It can also occur with a benign tumor of the parathyroid gland (located in the neck) called a parathyroid adenoma. Symptoms depend on the amount of calcium in blood and can vary from weakness, nausea, and thirst, to confusion, coma, and death. Hypercalcemia associated with malignant disease occurs most often with myeloma and with cancers of the prostate, breast, and lung. Treatment includes large doses of intravenous fluids, diuretics that increase urine flow, and the hormone calcitonin.

**hypernephroma** *See* Kidney Cancer (pages 173–174).

**hyperoxygenation** A technique that uses high-pressure oxygen to increase oxygen content in cancer cells, thereby making them more sensitive to radiation therapy. Hyperoxygenation is based upon the theory that a lack of oxygen is often the main cause of the failure of cancer to respond to radiation therapy.

**hyperplasia** Too much growth of cells or tissues in a specific area, such as the lining of the prostate. *See also* Benign Prostatic Hypertrophy.

**hypersplenism** A condition in which the spleen removes elements from the blood (red blood cells, white blood cells, platelets) at a faster-than-normal rate. Hypersplenism causes anemia, infection, and bleeding, respectively, and is often caused by leukemias and lymphoma involving the spleen. Splenectomy (surgical removal of the spleen) may be needed in severe cases.

**hyperthermia** A procedure for raising body temperature. It is used to increase the effects of chemotherapy and radiation therapy. Although hyperthermia may have a place in treating cancer, it is not used widely because of the numerous technical difficulties involved.

**hypoxic cell sensitizer** Chemical compounds, such as nitroimidazoles, that mimic hyperoxygenation (an increase in oxygen content) of tissues and make cancer cells more sensitive to radiation therapy. *See also* Nitroimidazole.

**hysterectomy** Removal of the uterus. This is used to treat endometrial and cervical cancers, and it is used together with oophorectomy to treat ovarian cancer. Although the operation can be done either through the abdomen (abdominal hysterectomy) or vagina (vaginal hysterectomy),when used for treating cancer it is usually done through the abdomen. *See also* Cervical Cancer (pages 161–163); Endometrial Cancer (pages 165–167); Ovarian Cancer (pages 190–191).

# I

℞ **ibuprofen** Also known by the trade names Motrin® and Advil®, this drug belongs to a group of drugs known as nonsteroidal anti-inflammatory drugs (NSAIDs). It is a nonopioid analgesic used as a pain reliever.

℞ **Idamycin®** *See* Idarubicin.

℞ **idarubicin** Also known by the trade name Idamycin®, this drug belongs to a group of drugs known as anthracycline antibiotics. It is primarily used to treat acute myelogenous leukemia.

℞ **idoxifene** This investigational drug belongs to a group of drugs known as antihormones. It is a synthetic antiestrogen and is being tested as a treatment for several types of cancer, including breast cancer.

℞ **Ifex®** *See* Ifosfamide.

℞ **ifosfamide** Also known by the trade name Ifex®, this alkylating type of chemotherapy drug is similar to cyclophosphamide. It is used to treat a variety of cancers including soft tissue sarcomas, germ cell testicular cancer, non-Hodgkin's lymphoma, and small cell lung cancer. The major adverse effect is hemorrhagic cystitis (severe bladder irritation with bleeding), which can be prevented by giving the drug mesna at the same time.

**ileal bladder** An artificial bladder fashioned from a portion of small intestine (ileum), which is used after cystectomy (removal of the bladder). It lies completely within the abdomen, with a self-sealing stoma (opening) in the skin through which urine is drained intermittently using a small catheter. The ileal bladder is a great advance in rehabilitating post-cystectomy patients by freeing them from wearing a bag to collect urine. *See also* Bladder Cancer (pages 154–156).

**ileostomy** An opening (stoma) created surgically between the skin and lower small intestine (ileum) through which bowel contents drain outside the body, which is needed after the entire colon and rectum are removed. A recent innovation (continent ileostomy) is a pouch or reservoir inside the abdomen, made from the ileum, which holds bowel material until drained with a catheter. It enables ileostomates (ileostomy patients) to not be required to wear a bag most of the time. *See also* Stoma.

℞ **Ilotycin®** *See* Erythromycin.

**imaging study** A diagnostic test that displays the structure and/or function of internal organs. It is indispensable in diagnosing cancer and determining the stage of malignant disease. Among the most available studies are diagnostic x-ray, CT, MRI, radioisotope scans, and ultrasonography. Positron emission tomography (PET) is a newer imaging study, which measures chemical reactions in the body and is available only in a few cancer centers and large hospitals.

℞ **imipenem/cilastatin sodium** Also known by the trade name Primaxin®, this drug is an antibiotic.

℞ **imipramine pamoate** Also known by the trade name Tofranil-PM®, this drug belongs to a group of drugs known as tricyclic antidepressants.

**immune response** The body's protective reaction to foreign substances (bacteria and viruses). It is generated by the immune system.

**immune system** A highly complex network of specialized cells and organs that produce the immune response to protect the body against outside invaders (bacteria, viruses, fungi, antigens), as well as malignant cells that arise in the body. Immunity, the condition of being protected, is provided by humoral immunity —protein particles in blood and lymph, such as antibodies; and cellular immunity—cells, including lymphocytes and macrophages that attack and destroy foreign substances. Immunotherapy is treatment using the body's immune system. *See also* Immunity; Immunotherapy.

**immunity** The situation or state of being protected from disease, which results from either previous infection or vaccination. Also, the body's response to a variety of antigens. *See also* Immune System.

**immunoglobulin** Any one of a group of related protein molecules found in serum (liquid portion that remains after the blood clots) that act as antibodies in the immune system. There are five different classes of immunoglobulins, known as IgG, IgM, IgE, IgA, and IgD, each with a different structure and function.

**immunosuppression** Interference or prevention of the body's immune (protective) response, which may result from diseases such as AIDS or drug treatment to prevent rejection of organ and tissue transplants.

**immunotherapy** Treatment using the body's immune (protective) system. Because cancer often results from failure of the immune system (as in AIDS and drug immunosuppression), substances that stimulate the body's natural defense system should affect (and hopefully destroy) malignancies.

Among the immunotherapy agents long used to treat malignant disease are BCG and levamasole. Today, tumor vaccines made from malignant cells are used to generate antibodies to various tumor antigens, notably melanoma. Newer immunotherapy agents such as cytokines, which are protein molecules (interferons and interleukins) produced by white blood cells and other cells, are being used against various tumors. Antibody produced by a clone or genetically similar cells (monoclonal antibody), which has an anticancer drug or radioisotopes attached, can enable chemotherapy and radiation to affect only the cancer whose antigen attaches to the antibody while sparing normal cells from the effects of chemotherapy and radiation. Also being studied are ways to induce T cell lymphocytes to more effectively attack malignancies. These include lymphokine-activated killer (LAK) cells and tumor-infiltrating lymphocytes (TIL).

Because many of the agents in cancer immunotherapy severely injure bone marrow, and cause flu-like symptoms including fever and muscle aches, research continues for immunotherapy that will have fewer adverse effects. *See also* Immune System.

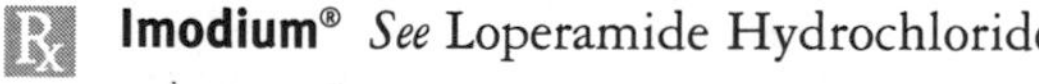

**Imodium®** *See* Loperamide Hydrochloride.

**implant** An artificial form used to restore the shape of an organ after surgery. *See also* Breast Implant.

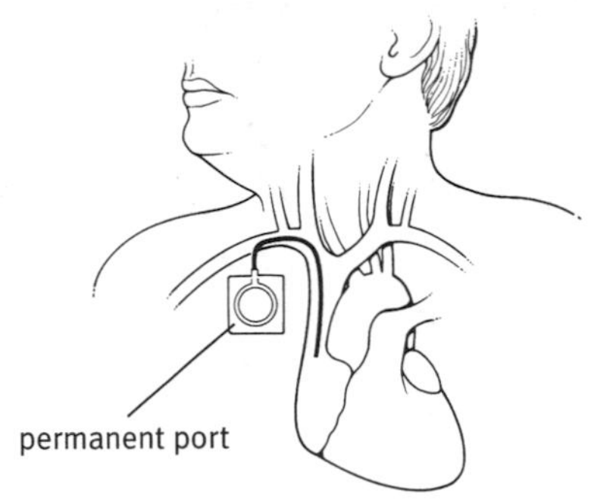


**implantable port** A device placed beneath the skin and connected to a vein, which enables cancer patients to receive intravenous (IV) medication and have blood sampled without repeated needle sticks of scarred and often hard-to-find veins. A needle puncture through the skin overlying the port provides access to a small plastic or metal chamber attached to a vein by a small plastic tube or catheter. The minor operation to place the device is usually done under local anesthesia. *See also* Vascular Access Device.

**impotence** Not being able to have or keep an erection of the penis.

**in situ cancer** *See* Carcinoma In Situ.

℞ **Inapsine®** *See* Droperidol.

**incidence** Used in statistical analysis to describe the number of specified new events (such as cancers) occurring in a certain group of people over a particular time.

**incision** A cut made during surgery.

**incisional biopsy** Removal of a portion of tissue for examination; often used during operations to diagnose and stage cancer. It must be done carefully to prevent spread of cancer cells. Also, the term to describe the tissue specimen removed during incisional biopsy. *See also* Biopsy.

**incontinence** Partial or complete loss of urinary or bowel control.

℞ **Indocin®** *See* Indomethacin.

℞ **indomethacin** Also known by the trade name Indocin®, this drug belongs to a group of drugs known as nonsteroidal anti-inflammatory drugs (NSAIDs). It is a nonopioid analgesic used as a pain reliever.

**infectious mononucleosis** A disease of sudden onset in young people and children due to the Epstein-Barr virus spread by saliva. It causes fever, sore throat, swollen lymph nodes, and enlarged spleen, which at first may be confused with lymphatic cancer (Hodgkin's disease, lymphomas). A positive blood test result for heterophile antibody confirms the diagnosis of mononucleosis. *See also* Epstein-Barr Virus.

**inferior vena cava** *See* Vena Cava.

**inflammation** The body's response to injury or stimulation from chemical, physical, or biologic (bacteria and fungus) substances. It involves different cells and chemical reactions in tissues that attempt to heal. The fundamental occurrences or signs associated with inflammation (not all of which are invariably present) are swelling, warmth, pain, redness, and often impaired function.

**inflammatory** Relating to inflammation.

**inflammatory bowel disease** Chronic ulcerative colitis (CUC) and Crohn's disease of the colon or rectum produce inflammation of the large intestine and cause severe swelling, ulcers, bleeding, infection, and pain in the colon and/or rectum. People with either disease (especially CUC) of long duration are at increased risk of colorectal cancer and should have regular colonoscopy to identify early colon and rectal tumors. Also, people with long-standing ulcerative colitis are at increased risk for developing sclerosing cholangitis (scaring of the bile ducts), which is often associated with bile duct cancer. *See also* Crohn's Disease; Ulcerative Colitis.

**inflammatory breast cancer** An uncommon, rapidly growing cancer that causes breast pain, swelling, redness, and warmth. It is easily confused with severe breast abscess (infection) and can only be diagnosed with a biopsy. In the past, this cancer was always fatal; but today, approximately one-third of women live for 10 or more years after receiving combined therapy with chemotherapy, radiation, and surgery.

**informed consent** The process by which patients or parents agree to treatment. A legal document that explains a course of treatment, the risks, benefits, and possible alternatives.

**infraclavicular nodes** Lymph nodes located beneath the clavicle (collarbone).

**inherited** Any characteristic that is passed from parent to offspring such as skin and eye color; and conditions such as color-blindness, multiple polyps, and medullary thyroid cancer. *See also* Heredity.

**injection** The introduction of a drug or other fluid through a needle; most often into the subcutaneous fatty tissue beneath the skin (subcutaneous), into the muscle (intramuscular), into a vein (intravenous), or into an artery (intra-arterial).

**inoperable** Indication that a condition, such as advanced-stage cancer, cannot be operated upon or cannot be relieved or removed by an operation.

**insulin** The hormone that lowers blood glucose (sugar). It is produced in pancreatic cells in the islets of Langerhans, groups of endocrine cells scattered throughout the pancreas.

**insulinoma** A rare, insulin-producing tumor of the pancreas, considered malignant only if spread beyond the pancreas. It results in low blood glucose (sugar) that causes weakness, trembling, sweating, confusion, and in extreme instances, coma and death.

℞ **interferon** Any one of a several related proteins (cytokines), including interferon-alpha (IFN-$\alpha$), interferon-beta (IFN-$\beta$), and interferon-gamma (IFN-$\gamma$), produced by white blood cells and other cells responding to viral infection and other antigens. All act against a variety of cancers, and IFN-$\alpha$ is used as immunotherapy of melanoma, hairy cell leukemia, Kaposi's sarcoma, and early bladder and cervical cancers.

℞ **interleukin** Any one of at least seven related proteins (cytokines) that stimulate cell growth and function as part of the body's immune (protective) mechanism. Interleukin-2 (IL-2) promotes growth of white blood cells, especially the T cell variety that destroys both bacteria and malignant cells, and is being investigated as immunotherapy in advanced-stage melanoma and kidney cancer. *See* Oprelvekin.

**intermittent hormone therapy** A type of prostate cancer treatment in which hormonal drugs are stopped after a man's blood PSA level decreases to a very low level and remains stable for a while. If the PSA level begins to increase, the drugs are started again.

**internal mammary nodes** Lymph nodes beneath the breast bone on each side. Some breast cancers may spread to these nodes.

**intestinal polyposis** *See* Familial Adenomatous Polyposis.

**intestine** The tube-like passage from the stomach to the anus. It includes the small intestine (duodenum, jejunum, ileum), which absorbs digested food, nutrients, and liquids; and the large intestine (colon, rectum), which absorbs water and stores waste matter. Although the large intestine is frequently the site of cancer, the small intestine is rarely the origin of malignant tumors. Also called bowel. *See also* Duodenum; Jejunum.

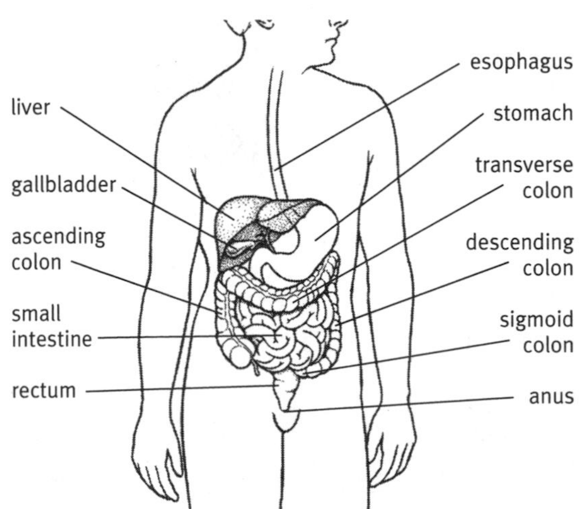


**intracranial pressure** Pressure within the skull; from fluid surrounding the brain and spinal cord largely produced in an area of the brain (cerebral ventricles). Increased pressure is caused by brain tumors, cancer spread to the brain, and head injury. Severe headache, nausea and vomiting, seizures, weakness, and disturbances of speech and sight are indications of increased pressure—a medical emergency that without prompt treatment can cause death. If a brain tumor cannot be removed, cortisone-like drugs such as dexamethasone that reduce brain inflammation, and diuretics such as mannitol that remove fluid from the brain are used to lower the pressure within the skull. *See also* Brain Tumor (pages 157–159).

**intraductal papillomas** Small, benign (noncancerous) polyp-like growths in the breast ducts that may cause a bloody discharge from the nipple. These are found mostly in women 45 to 50 years of age. If a woman has many papillomas, the risk of breast cancer is slightly increased. *See also* Breast Cancer (pages 159–161).

**intramuscular (IM)** Denoting something within a muscle; often used to describe the route by which a drug solution or other liquid is given (IM morphine).

**intraocular melanoma** *See* Uveal Melanoma.

**intravenous (IV)** Within a vein; often used to describe a needle or catheter (small tube) placed into a vein to deliver fluid. Also used to describe a particular drug administered by vein. Medication given intravenously takes effect rapidly and usually requires smaller doses than when given by injection (intramuscular or subcutaneous).

**intravenous pyelography** *See* Pyelography.

**invasion** Spread of cancer to surrounding structures, organs, or tissue either by growth into or destruction of adjacent tissue. In some cases, very early cancer (carcinoma in situ or preinvasive cancer) precedes invasive tumor.

**invasive cancer** Cancer involving adjacent tissue (most often the lining or mucosa of an organ) that is likely to metastasize (spread) to the lymph nodes and other sites. *See also* Carcinoma In Situ.

**invasive mole** *See* Chorioadenoma Destruens

**investigational** Under study; often used to described drugs used in clinical trials before they are approved for specific indications by the US Food and Drug Administration.

**iodine** A nonmetallic, chemical element having several radioactive forms (radioisotopes); used for both diagnosing and treating cancer. Iodine 123 (I-123) is used in thyroid scans, I-125 in small metal "seeds" is used in radiation therapy of prostate and lung cancers, and I-131 is used to diagnose and treat thyroid cancer.

**ionizing radiation** Radiation having sufficient energy to cause irradiated material to develop ions (atoms or groups of atoms with a positive (+) or negative (-) electrical charge). It is the type of radiation most often used to treat cancer, and is implied in terms such as radiation therapy, radiation treatment, etc. Ionizing radiation comes from machines (linear accelerator), natural radioactive elements (radium, radon), and human-made radioisotopes (cobalt, gold, iodine, iridium). *See also* Radiation Therapy.

**iridium** A silvery metal; the radioactive form (radioisotope I-192) is used in radiation therapy (brachytherapy) of cancer by placing (after loading) iridium wires in needles or plastic tubes previously inserted in or near a tumor. *See also* Brachytherapy; Radiation Therapy.

Rx **irinotecan** Also known by the trade name Camptosar®, this drug is the first new chemotherapy agent approved in the past 40 years for treating colon and rectal cancers. It is used for cancer that persists or recurs after prior treatment with fluorouracil (5-FU). It also shows promise in treating cancers of the cervix, ovary, and lung. The main adverse effects are diarrhea that may be severe, nausea, and decreased numbers of white blood cells.

**irradiate** To apply radiation; most often ionizing radiation used in cancer therapy. *See also* Ionizing Radiation; Radiation Therapy.

**islet cell** Any one of several different hormone-producing cells (alpha, beta, delta) present in small groups (islets of Langerhans) scattered throughout the pancreas. Among the hormones produced are glucagon (alpha cells) that raises blood sugar, insulin (beta cells) that lowers blood sugar, and somatostatin (delta cells) that inhibits other hormones including insulin.

**islet cell cancer** Malignant endocrine cancer of islet cells of the pancreas that includes insulinoma (beta cells), glucagonoma (alpha cells), and somatostatinoma (delta cells).

**isolated regional perfusion** A technique for giving high-dose intra-arterial chemotherapy in an arm or leg after blood vessels to the limb have been isolated from the remainder of the circulatory system. Keeping drugs from the remainder of the body protects bone marrow and other organs from high-dose chemotherapy. Although the procedure has long been used to treat advanced melanoma and sarcoma, it is not widely used, because it is both cumbersome and time-consuming. *See also* Chemotherapy.

**isotope** *See* Radioisotope.

℞ **itraconazole** Also known by the trade name Sporanox®, this drug is an antifungal agent that is used to treat severe infections.

**IVP** *See* Pyelography.

# J

**jaundice** Yellow discoloration of the skin and eyes, often associated with dark (cola-colored) urine; due to increased bile in blood and body tissues. When it occurs without abdominal pain, it is often the first symptom of cancers of the liver, biliary tract, or head of the pancreas, which block the flow of bile from the liver. Chemotherapy with fluorouracil (5-FU) and FUDR® given in the hepatic artery (artery to the liver) can also cause jaundice.

**jejunostomy** An opening into the jejunum, the mid-portion of the small intestine; most often a stoma (opening) created between the skin and jejunum to provide liquid nourishment for those unable to swallow. Today, it is often easily done with gastroscopy under local anesthetic. *See also* Stoma.

**jejunum** Mid-portion of the small intestine, located between the duodenum and ileum. *See also* Small Intestine Cancer (pages 201–202).

# K

℞ **kanamycin sulfate** Also known by the trade name Kantrex®, this is an antibiotic that belongs to a group of drugs known as aminoglycosides.

℞ **Kantrex®** *See* Kanamycin Sulfate.

**Kaposi's sarcoma** A cancer primarily of skin that also affects lymph nodes and internal organs. It was first noted as a skin tumor below the knee in elderly men of Jewish or Mediterranean origin in the United States and Europe. Today, three other types are recognized: a variety associated with people having organ transplant who receive drugs to suppress the immune system and prevent rejection, an AIDS-associated type similar to that seen in transplant patients, and a rapidly growing variety in African natives. *See also* Acquired Immunodeficiency Syndrome; Sarcoma; Skin Cancer (pages 199–201); Soft Tissue Cancer (pages 202–204).

℞ **Kefzol®** *See* Cefazolin Sodium.

**keratosis** A common benign (noncancerous) skin growth, mainly of two varieties: *seborrheic* keratosis, which never becomes cancer, occurs in middle age as a sharply outlined, dark brown wart-like growth on the skin; *actinic* keratosis, which may lead to skin cancer (squamous carcinoma), is a brown or black, raised, scaly, rough, growth in light-skinned people on sun-exposed areas. Because 25% of actinic keratoses become malignant, they should be removed or destroyed by electrocautery (electric current), cryotherapy (freezing), or chemotherapy (fluorouracil liquid or cream). *See also* Skin Cancer (pages 199–201).

℞ **ketoconazole** Also known by the trade name Nizoral®, this drug is an antifungal agent. It also slows the growth of prostate cancer and is sometimes used for advanced prostate cancer that has stopped reponding to hormonal therapy.

℞ **ketorolac tromethamine** Also known by the trade name Toradol®, this drug belongs to a group of drugs known as nonsteroidal anti-inflammatory drugs (NSAIDs). It is a nonopioid analgesic used as a pain reliever.

**kidney function study** A test to determine the ability of the kidneys to remove waste products from the blood. Increased amounts of the compounds creatinine and urea nitrogen (BUN) in blood indicate renal (kidney) failure, and a detailed study (creatinine clearance) measures the degree of failure. Renal failure can also result from cancer blocking urine flow from the kidneys, or the toxic effects of chemotherapy drugs on the kidneys, notably cis-platinum. *See also* Kidney Cancer (pages 173–174).

**Klatskin tumor** Bile duct cancer at or near the junction of the left and right bile ducts below the liver, where they join to form the common duct. *See also* Bile Duct Cancer (pages 153–154).

**Klinefelter's syndrome** A rare condition in males caused by an extra X chromosome (XXY), which results in high-pitched voice, enlarged breasts, and small testes. Individuals with this condition are more likely (than normal males) to develop breast cancer, leukemia, and germ cell tumor in the chest.

℞ **Klonopin®** *See* Clonazepam.

℞ **Kytril®** *See* Granisetron Hydrochloride.

# L

℞ **lactulose** Also known by the trade name Cholac®, this drug is used as a laxative. It is a very concentrated form of sugar.

**laparoscope** A lighted, magnifying instrument connected to a television monitor and used to examine the interior of the abdomen (abdominal cavity).

**laparoscopy** The surgical procedure using a laparoscope to biopsy suspected tumors and perform operations including gallbladder removal and appendectomy without opening the abdomen. Although laparoscopy requires general anesthesia, it is safe, well-tolerated, and less painful than laparotomy (abdominal surgery). In some instances laparoscopy is done as outpatient surgery.

**laparotomy** The general term to describe a surgical procedure that opens the abdomen; also used to diagnose and determine the extent (stage) of cancers in the abdomen. Although previously advised in almost all cases of Hodgkin's disease, it is used today only for selected patients. In some instances, laparotomy may be replaced by laparoscopy, a less involved procedure.

**large bowel cancer** *See* Colorectal Cancer (pages 163–165).

**large cell carcinoma** The least common variety of non-small cell lung cancer (NSLC), which accounts for 10% to 20% of malignant tumors originating in the lung. *See also* Lung Cancer (pages 180–182); Non-Small Cell Lung Cancer.

**laryngeal** Pertaining to the larynx (voice box). *See also* Laryngeal Cancer (pages 175–176).

**laryngectomy** Complete or partial removal of the larynx (voice box); used to treat laryngeal cancer. Total laryngectomy requires rehabilitation to restore the voice, and in many cases, esophageal speech or tracheoesophageal puncture (TEP) enables postlaryngectomy patients to speak without a vibrating instrument pressed against the neck. *See also* Laryngeal Cancer (pages 175–176).

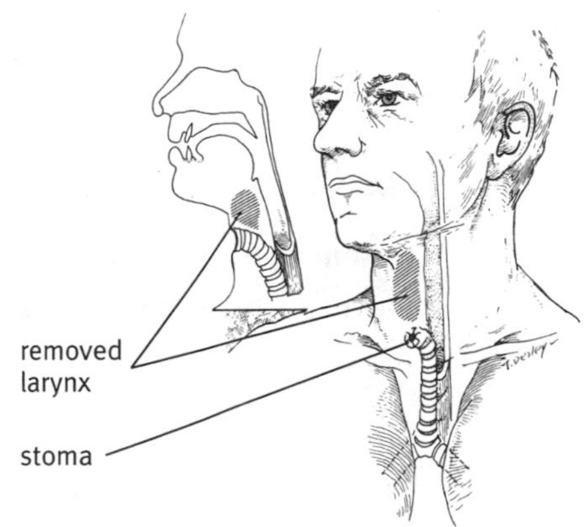


Illustration used by permission of the Mayo Foundation. From *Looking Forward...A Guidebook for the Laryngectomee,* by R.L. Keith, et al, New York, Theime-Stratton, Inc., and copyrighted by the Mayo foundation, 1984.

**laryngoscope** A lighted, magnifying instrument; used to examine and biopsy the larynx (voice box).

**laryngoscopy** The procedure to view and biopsy the interior of the larynx (voice box) and vocal cords using a laryngoscope passed down the throat under local anesthesia.

**larynx** A complex organ in the neck made up of several cartilages and moveable elastic tissues, which produces the voice, prevents swallowed material from entering the lung, and enables coughing. Also called the voice box. *See also* Laryngeal Cancer (pages 175–176).

**laser** A device (light amplification by stimulated emission of radiation) that produces a concentrated, intense, narrow beam of light, whose wavelength varies according to the light source (argon, carbon dioxide, neodymium). Lasers are used to treat carcinoma in situ and early-stage tumors of larynx and cervix, palliate brain tumors, and relieve obstruction caused by advanced esophageal and rectal cancers. This device is also used in flow cytometry.

**latissimus dorsi flap procedure** A method of breast reconstruction that uses the long flap muscle of the back by rotating it to the chest area.

℞ **Laudanum®** *See* Deodorized Tincture of Opium.

**leiomyosarcoma** An uncommon cancer of smooth or involuntary muscle (muscle not under conscious control). This cancer, a variety of soft tissue sarcoma, can arise in any location, but most often occurs in the peritoneum (tissue that lines the abdominal cavity) and retroperitoneum (space behind the abdomen), where it can grow to a very large size. In the skin, it most often occurs as multiple small lumps. It can also develop from the muscular walls of the uterus. Rarely, tumor can involve blood vessels (pulmonary artery, inferior vena cava) and obstruct the flow of blood. Surgical removal is the mainstay of treatment. *See also* Sarcoma; Soft Tissue Cancer (pages 202–204).

**lentigo maligna** *See* Melanoma (pages 182–184).

**lesion** Any unnatural or abnormal change in the body that can be seen, felt, or identified by means of imaging studies such as x-ray, ultrasonography, CT, and MRI.

℞ **letrozole** Also known by the trade name Femara®, this drug, similar to anastrozole, is used in hormone therapy of recurrent breast cancer in postmenopasual women previously treated with either tamoxifen or toremifene.

℞ **leucovorin** Also known as folinic acid or citrovorum factor, this is a chemical compound used to counteract the effects of high-dose methotrexate used in treating osteosarcoma. It also increases the effects of fluorouracil (5-FU) in treating colon cancer patients with adjuvant therapy and with advanced (stage III) colorectal cancer. It can be given by mouth, artery, or vein, and its adverse effects include thrombocytosis (an increased number of platelets in the blood), diarrhea, skin rash, and itching.

℞ **Leukeran®** *See* Chlorambucil.

℞ **Leukine®** *See* Sargramostim.

**leukocoria** A large white spot in the pupil, due to light reflecting from a tumor deep within the eye. It is most often caused by retinoblastoma, the most common malignant eye tumor in children. Also called cat eye reflex. *See also* Retinoblastoma (pages 196–197).

**leukocyte** *See* White Blood Cell.

**leukocytosis** Having more than the usual number of white blood cells.

**leukopenia** The condition in which the number of white blood cells (leukocytes) is decreased in blood. *See* Granulocytopenia.

**leukoplakia** A flat, white patch on the lip or inside the mouth that cannot be wiped off; the precursor of a type of cancer, squamous cell carcinoma. It also occurs on the genitals in women. Treatment is either limited surgical removal, or destruction by cryotherapy (freezing), electrocautery (electric current), or laser.

℞ **leuprolide** Also known by the trade name Lupron®, this is an injectable, synthetic hormone given daily to treat the symptoms of advanced prostate cancer. It is also used in place of orchiectomy (removal of the testicles) and estrogen therapy. It lowers the level of male hormone from the testicles (testosterone) that controls the growth of both normal and cancerous prostate tissue. During the first week it may cause a flare (temporary increase in bone pain).

℞ **Leustatin®** *See* Cladribine.

℞ **levamisole** Also known by the trade name Ergamisol®, this oral drug is used in the immunotherapy of colon cancer spread to lymph nodes. Initially developed to treat animal parasites, it is given with intravenous (IV) fluorouracil (5-FU) to increase the likelihood of cure following surgery in those with lymph node metastasis. It may also be useful in treating melanoma.

℞ **Levaquin®** *See* Levofloxacin.

**LeVeen shunt** The original device contained entirely in the body to relieve ascites (fluid buildup in the abdomen) due to cancer. It has three parts: a tube placed in the abdomen, a smaller tube inserted in a jugular vein (neck vein), and a one-way valve in between. Pressing on the valve beneath the skin pumps ascitic fluid into the blood circulation, from which it is removed by the kidneys. Both the LeVeen shunt and a newer device (the Denver® shunt) control ascites without repeated needle drainage that depletes the body of protein-rich ascitic fluid. *See also* Ascites; Denver® Shunt; Paracentesis; Shunt.

℞ **Levo-Dromoran®** *See* Levorphanol Tartrate.

℞ **levofloxacin** Also known by the trade name Levaquin®, this drug is an antibiotic that belongs to a group of drugs known as fluoroquinolones.

℞ **levorphanol tartrate** Also known by the trade name Levo-Dromoran®, this drug is a synthetic opioid analgesic used as a pain reliever.

**LHRH** Abbreviation for **l**euteinizing **h**ormone-**r**eleasing **h**ormone, a hormone produced by the hypothalamus, which is a tiny gland in the brain.

**Li-Fraumeni cancer syndrome** *See* Cancer Family Syndrome.

℞ **lidocaine** Also known by the trade name Xylocaine®, this anesthetic drug is injected in the skin or around nerves to prevent or relieve pain. Viscous Xylocaine, a thick, flavored mouth rinse, is used to relieve mouth and throat pain caused by irritation or dryness resulting from chemotherapy or radiation therapy to the head and neck.

**limited breast surgery** Limited breast surgery removes the breast cancer and a small amount of tissue around the cancer, but preserves most of the breast. Also called lumpectomy; sequential excision; tylectomy. *See also* Breast Cancer (pages 159–161).

℞ **linezolid** Also known by the trade name Zyvox®, this drug is an antibiotic that belongs to a group of drugs called oxazolidinones, a new class of antibiotics. It is used to treat bacterial infections that are resistant to other antibiotics.

**liposarcoma** A cancer that arises in fat; a variety of soft tissue sarcoma found most often in adults between the ages of 50 and 60. It varies from a slow growing variety (well-differentiated) that never metastasizes (spreads), to a type that quickly spreads (pleomorphic), especially to the lungs. The tumor is found most often in the retroperitoneal space behind the abdomen and in the muscles deep in the thigh. It occasionally occurs as multiple tumors. *See also* Retroperitoneum; Sarcoma; Soft Tissue Cancer (pages 202–204).

℞ **liposomal tretinoin** Also known by the trade name Atragen®, this drug causes acute promyelocytic leukemia (APL) cells to mature, thus causing them to stop dividing. Incorporation of this drug in a liposome (fat molecule) allows it to be given intravenously so that blood levels may be higher for a longer time. It is being studied in patients newly diagnosed with acute promyelocytic leukemia, Kaposi's sarcoma, and other types of cancer.

**liver fluke** Any one of several worm-like internal parasites associated with bile duct cancer and cholangiocarcinoma (liver cancer) in East Asia. Taken into the body in raw or partially cooked, contaminated fish and shellfish, the parasite finds its way to bile ducts where it causes cholangitis (persistent or chronic irritation) that gives rise to cancer. *See also* Bile Duct Cancer (pages 153–154); Liver Cancer (pages 178–179).

**liver function tests** Several blood tests (bilirubin, alkaline phosphatase, albumin) taken together to indicate activity (function) of the liver; used to detect cancer in the liver, as well as bile duct and pancreatic cancers that obstruct bile flow from the liver. *See also* Bile Duct Cancer (pages 153–154); Liver Cancer (pages 178–179); Pancreatic Cancer (pages 191–193).

**liver scan** An imaging study of the liver, that uses radioactive material absorbed by the liver. After the radioisotope is given intravenously, a device (gamma camera) to detect radiation is moved over the abdomen. Both benign liver tumors and liver cancers do not absorb radioactive material and appear as white (cold) spots on the x-ray film. *See also* Imaging Study; Liver Cancer (pages 178–179).

**lobe** A natural, anatomic subdivision of an organs such as the lungs, liver, thyroid, brain, or prostate.

**lobectomy** Surgical removal of a lobe; used for cancers of the thyroid, liver, and lung to remove tumor confined to a lobe of the organ.

**lobular carcinoma in situ (LCIS)** The earliest (noninvasive) stage of breast cancer that arises in milk-producing glands. Because it cannot be felt, LCIS is discovered during mammography or biopsy for some other breast problem, usually benign fibrocystic disease. The lesion is considered a "marker" that indicates breast cancer is more likely to occur in either breast in the future. The usual treatment advised for lobular carcinoma in situ is careful follow-up with frequent re-examinations to detect early cancer. Tamoxifen may also be advised. *See also* Appendix for Cancer Detection Guidelines; Breast Cancer (pages 159–161).

**lobules** The glands in a woman's breasts that produce milk.

**localized cancer** A cancer that is confined to the place where it started; that is, it has not spread to distant parts of the body.

℞ **Lomotil®** *See* Diphenoxylate Hydrochloride and Atropine.

℞ **lomustine** *See* Nitrosourea.

℞ **loperamide hydrochloride** Also known by the trade name Imodium®, this drug is an antidiarrheal agent that belongs to the group of drugs known as piperidine derivatives.

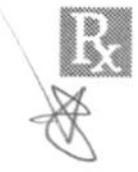

**lorazepam** Also known by the trade name Ativan®, this is an anxiolytic (anxiety reliever) drug that belongs to a group of drugs known as benzodiazepines. It is also used in the management of nausea and vomiting associated with cancer chemotherapy.

**L-PAM®** *See* Melphalan Hydrochloride.

**lumbar puncture** Needle puncture of the lower spine to sample and measure the pressure of spinal fluid—the colorless watery fluid produced in the brain and surrounding the brain and spinal cord.

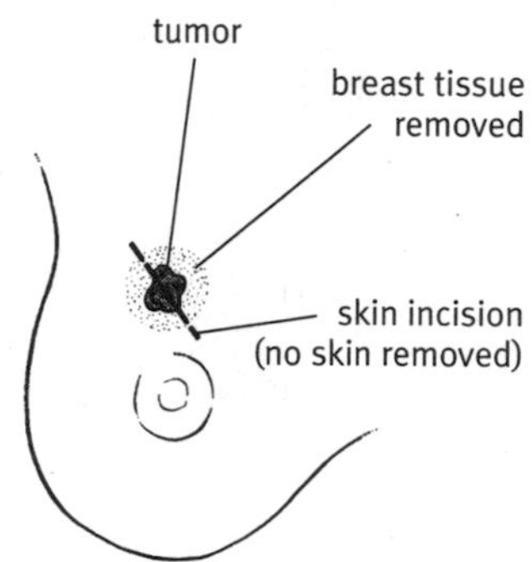


**lumpectomy** Surgical removal of a lump or swollen area. Most often used to describe the operation to remove a breast cancer in which only the tumor and a narrow rim of surrounding breast tissue are removed. Lumpectomy has replaced mastectomy (removal of the entire breast) as the usual operation for most breast cancers. It is usually followed by radiation therapy to the breast to prevent a recurrence in the breast. *See also* Breast Cancer (pages 159–161); Limited Breast Surgery.

**Lupron®** *See* Leuprolide.

**lycopenes** Vitamin-like antioxidants that help prevent damage to DNA. People who have diets rich in tomatoes, which contain lycopene, appear to have a lower risk of certain types of cancer, especially cancers of the prostate, lung, and stomach. Further research is needed to determine what role, if any, lycopene has in the prevention or treatment of cancer. Found in tomatoes, grapefruit, and watermelon.

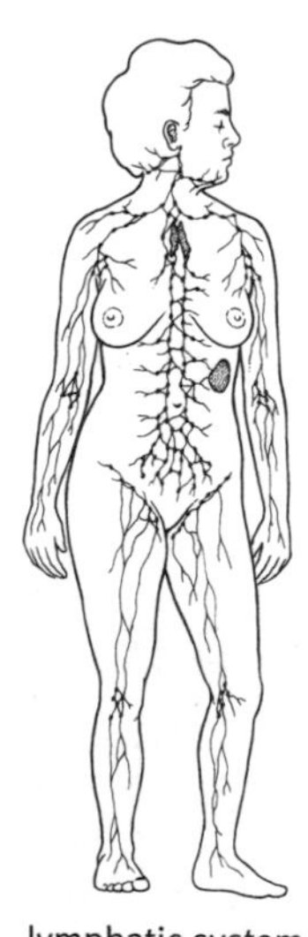
lymphatic system

**lymph** Clear, watery fluid that contains varying numbers of white blood cells, and few red blood cells. It collects from tissue and circulates through lymph channels to lymph nodes. Metastasis (spread of cancer) frequently occurs from cancer cells passing through lymph channels to adjacent (regional) lymph nodes.

**lymph node** Any one of hundreds of bean-shaped structures made up of lymphocytes, a type of white blood cell (leukocyte). A part of the immune system that protects the body from infection. Lymph nodes are found throughout the body, especially under arms (axillary nodes), in groins (inguinal nodes), along the sides of the neck (cervical nodes), and adjacent to internal organs. Nodal swelling occurs either from cancer or noncancerous disease and from infection. Although cancer in a lymph node is most often spread from a malignant tumor in an adjacent organ, it may result from cancer arising in the node, such as in Hodgkin's disease, leukemia, or lymphoma. Lymph node biopsy is used to diagnose and determine the extent (stage) of cancer, and either lymphadenectomy (surgical removal) or radiation therapy is the usual treatment for adjacent (regional) lymph nodes involved with cancer from some other site.

**lymphadenectomy** Surgical removal of lymph node(s). Removal of adjacent (regional) lymph nodes together with the organ or site involved with cancer has been the time-honored operation for treating most malignant tumors. Therapeutic lymphadenectomy removes only enlarged adjacent (regional) nodes assumed to contain cancer, and prophylactic lymphadenectomy removes adjacent nodes, irrespective of whether they appear involved. Today, the frequent use of postoperative chemotherapy and radiation therapy to nodes adjacent to a tumor (as in breast cancer) has brought into question the need for the routine removal of regional lymph nodes. For melanoma (and increasingly, breast cancer) with no obvious spread to lymph nodes, identifying and biopsying the node(s) closest to tumor (sentinel node) makes lymphadenectomy necessary only if cancer cells are found in the sentinel node. However, removal of a few nodes adjacent to a cancer is necessary to accurately stage most malignancies.

**lymphangiogram** The image obtained by lymphangiography.

**lymphangiography** A radiology procedure which outlines lymph nodes and lymphatic tissue and is most often used to evaluate retroperitoneal nodes (abdominal lymph nodes adjacent to the spine) in staging Hodgkin's disease and lymphoma. Dye that is opaque to x-rays is injected into lymph channels in the foot, after which x-ray pictures (lymphangiograms) are made of the abdomen. It is being used less frequently today than in the past since we have better tests such as MRI and CT scan to examine the areas in question. *See also* Imaging Study.

**lymphatic** Pertaining to lymph.

**lymphedema** Painless swelling most often in fatty subcutaneous tissue beneath the skin in an arm or leg; due to the accumulation of lymph (fluid). It occurs most often after inguinal lymphadenectomy (removal of lymph nodes in the groin) or axillary lymphadenectomy (removal of lymph nodes under the arm) and sometimes from cancer blocking the flow of lymph.

**lymphocyte** A variety of white blood cell, or leukocyte, which evolves from a primitive cell (stem cell) originating in the bone marrow. Stem cells that develop into white blood cells in the thymus are T cell (thymus-derived) lymphocytes, and those that mature into white blood cells in bone marrow are B cell lymphocytes. Both cell types function as part of the body's immune (protective) mechanism by spreading through blood and lymph to different sites in the body, including lymph nodes, spleen, tonsils, throat (Waldeyer's ring); small intestine (Peyer's patches). Lymphocytes are not present in the brain and spinal cord (central nervous) system. *See also* B Cell; T Cell; White Blood Cell.

**lymphocytic** Having to do with lymphocytes, a type of white blood cell (WBC).

**lymphokine-activated killer (LAK) cells** Lymphocytes grown in the laboratory that are able to kill some cancer cells. They are produced by exposing lymphocytes, a variety of white blood cell (leukocyte), to relatively high doses of the cytokine interleukin-2 (IL-2). LAK cells are being studied as immunotherapy for many different cancers, including melanoma and leukemia.

**lymphoma** *See* Hodgkin's Disease (pages 172–173); Non-Hodgkin's Lymphoma (pages 188–190).

**Lynch cancer syndrome** Either of two cancer family syndromes in which family members have a high likelihood of developing either of two malignant disease states. Lynch Type I is colorectal cancer not associated with multiple intestinal polyposis; Lynch Type II is predominantly colorectal, endometrial, ovarian, and less often stomach and other cancers. *See also* Cancer Family Syndrome.

# M

**macrophage** A type of white blood cell that engulfs foreign material.

℞ **MagCitrate®** *See* Magnesium Citrate.

℞ **magnesium citrate** Also known by the trade name MagCitrate®, this drug is a saline laxative used to treat constipation.

**magnetic resonance imaging (MRI)** Magnetic resonance imaging is the technique that makes cross-sectional and three-dimensional pictures of the body without the use of x-rays. It is widely used in staging cancer because of the very detailed pictures it produces. Although MRI is painless, some older machines may be confining, especially to children. Because a strong magnetic field is produced, people with implanted metal devices (cardiac pace makers, heart valves), which could be dislodged cannot be imaged. *See also* Imaging Study.

**malignancy** The condition or property of being malignant. It is most often used to indicate cancer. *See also* Neoplasm; Tumor.

**malignant** Anything that resists therapy, and without immediate treatment is likely to become worse and possibly fatal. When used to describe a tumor, it denotes cancer that has the ability to invade (grow into) adjacent tissue and metastasize (spread) to lymph nodes, and distant sites and organs. *See also* Cancerous.

**malignant fibrous histiocytoma (MFH)** The most common soft tissue tumor of the arms and legs, and rare in bone. It most often affects adults between the ages of 60 to 70, although it may occur earlier. MFH presents as a painless mass or lump in the leg, and less often, in the arm. *See also* Sarcoma; Soft Tissue Cancer (pages 202–204).

**malignant pleural effusion** *See* Effusion.

**mammogram** The image or picture produced by mammography. The American Cancer Society recommends screening mammograms once yearly beginning at age 40, but they may be indicated at an earlier age. *See also* Appendix for Cancer Detection Guidelines; Breast Cancer (pages 159–161).

**mammography** A study of the breast to obtain images (mammograms). It is invaluable for diagnosing tumors too small to feel and for positioning biopsy needles in small breast lesions. The amount of radiation from mammography is negligible, and for most women the procedure is relatively painless. There are two types of mammograms: screening and diagnostic. Screening mammograms are performed in women who have no clinical evidence or suspicion of a lump or cancer; diagnostic mammograms are done when there is a suspected abnormality in the breast or to obtain special views of the breast for other reasons. *See also* Breast Cancer (pages 159–161); Digital Mammography.

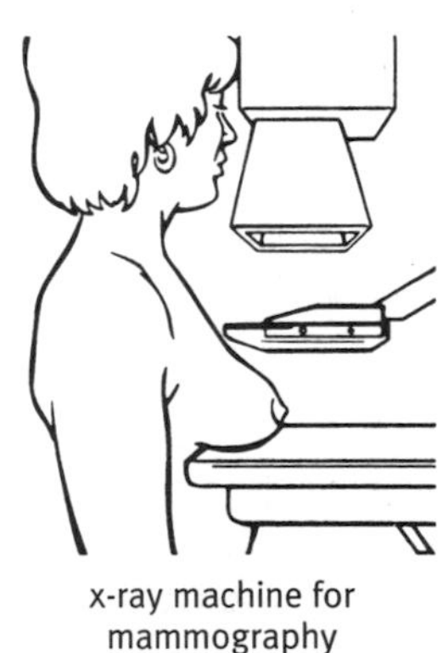

x-ray machine for mammography

**mammoplasty** Plastic surgery used to reconstruct the breast or to change the shape, size, or position of the breast. Reduction mammoplasty reduces the size of the breast. Augmentation mammoplasty enlarges a woman's breasts, usually with implants. Mammoplasty also applies to the surgical procedure to reconstruct the breast after more radical breast surgery. *See also* Breast Cancer (pages 159–161); Breast Reconstruction.

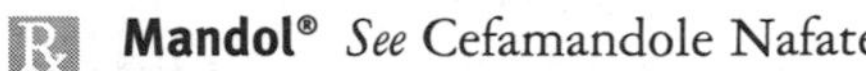

℞ **Mandol®** *See* Cefamandole Nafate.

℞ **mannitol** Also known by the trade name Osmitrol®, this is a diuretic drug that increases urine output from the kidneys by drawing fluid from tissues. It is used to prevent kidney injury from cisplatin, bladder injury (cystitis) from cyclophosphamide, and reduce brain swelling from brain tumors and cancer spread to the brain. *See also* Diuretic; Furosemide.

**margin** Edge of the tissue removed during surgery. A negative surgical margin is a sign that no cancer was left behind. A positive surgical margin indicates that cancer cells were found at the outer edge of the tissue removed and is usually a sign that some cancer remains in the body.

℞ **Marinol®** *See* Dronabinol.

**mastectomy** Removal of the entire breast, which usually includes the skin and nipple; used to treat breast cancer. Radical mastectomy also removes the two chest muscles beneath the breast (pectoralis major and minor) and lymph nodes under the arm (axially nodes). Today, radical surgery is seldom indicated except for advanced cancers, including the ones involving underlying muscle. Modified radical mastectomy preserves the pectoralis major muscle and is less likely to cause lymphedema (swelling of the arm) than does radical mastectomy. It is often advised for women with small breasts in whom a breast sparing procedure (lumpectomy) would leave a sizable deformity; and for women who do not wish a breast sparing procedure that necessitates postoperative radiation to the breast. Total (simple) mastectomy that leaves the muscles and lymph nodes intact, and partial mastectomy that removes only part of the breast are advised when lumpectomy cannot completely remove a cancer. *See also* Breast Cancer (pages 159–161); Breast Implant; Breast Reconstruction; Lymphedema.

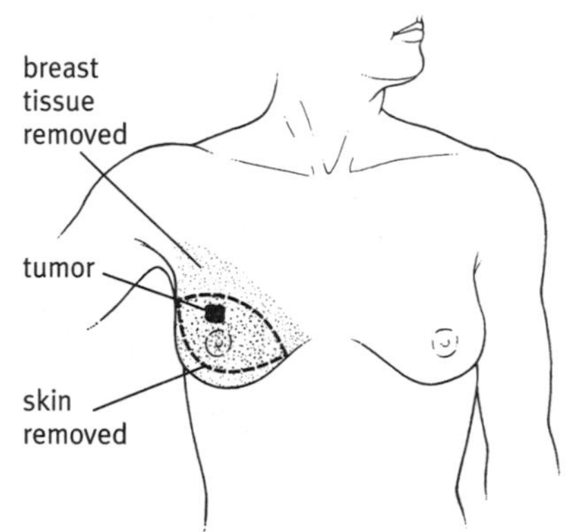


**mastitis** Inflammation or infection of the breast.

℞ **Matulane®** *See* Procarbazine Hydrochloride.

℞ **Maxipime®** *See* Cefepime.

℞ **MeCCNU®** *See* Methyl-CCNU and Nitrosourea.

℞ **mechlorethamine hydrochloride** Also known as nitrogen mustard and by the trade name Mustargen®, this was the first chemical compound specifically used to treat cancer, and the forerunner of all cytotoxic chemotherapy agents (drugs that kill cancer cells). Today, this alkylating type of anticancer agent is used mainly to treat Hodgkin's disease and lymphoma. Adverse effects include nausea and vomiting, and bone marrow injury.

**mediastinoscope** A lighted instrument (endoscope) to view and biopsy the mediastinum (middle of the chest).

**mediastinoscopy** The procedure done under general anesthesia using a mediastinoscope to diagnose and stage malignancies in the chest (lung cancer, Hodgkin's disease, lymphoma) and to identify chest diseases such as sarcoidosis, a benign but potentially life threatening inflammation in the central chest area.

**mediastinum** The middle of the chest in front of the spine that contains thoracic (chest) organs other than the lungs. These include: heart and large blood vessels (aorta, superior and inferior vena cava, pulmonary arteries and veins), windpipe or trachea, esophagus, thymus, and lymph nodes.

**medulla** The central or inner part of an organ. In the adrenal glands, the adrenal medulla produces the hormones epinephrine and norepinephrine. The medulla oblongata is part of the brain between the lower part of the brain (brain stem) and spinal cord.

**medullary carcinoma** Two distinct cancers having nothing in common but their name. Medullary breast carcinoma is an uncommon malignancy with a more favorable outlook than most other breast cancers.

Medullary thyroid carcinoma is a cancer that produces the hormone calcitonin. *See also* Thyroid Cancer (pages 207–209).

**medulloblastoma** A variety of brain tumor that affects both children and young adults. Unlike other tumors of the brain, it is capable of spreading outside the skull to bone and other organs. Although the tumor is very responsive to both radiation therapy and chemotherapy, only about half of the patients are cured. *See also* Brain Tumor (pages 157–159).

℞ **Mefoxin®** *See* Cefoxitin Sodium.

℞ **Megace®** *See* Megestrol.

℞ **megestrol** Also known by the trade name Megace®, this is a synthetic hormone similar to naturally-occurring progesterone produced by the ovary and placenta (afterbirth); used to treat advanced endometrial and breast cancers. It is also of benefit in improving nutrition and promoting weight gain in cancer patients.

**melena** Passage of a black, tar-like bowel movement due to blood in the gastrointestinal (GI) tract exposed to digestive juices (bile, pancreatic juice, stomach acid); sometimes the first indication of cancer of the stomach. *See also* Stomach Cancer (pages 204–206).

**melphalan hydrochloride** Also known as L-phenylalanine mustard (L-PAM®) and by the trade name Alkeran®, this is an alkylating chemotherapy drug used in treating different malignancies, primarily malignant myeloma. It significantly increases the risk of developing unrelated cancer, particularly acute leukemia.

**MEN** *See* Multiple Endocrine Neoplasia.

**menarche** The time of the first menstrual period, which today in American girls is occurring at an earlier age (11–12 years). This is probably due to improved nutrition, and the absence of childhood illness. Early onset of menstruation has been used to explain the increasing occurrence of breast cancer in American women. Girls who do not begin menstruation until the late teens have less risk for developing breast later in life.

**meningioma** A common type of brain tumor of the meninges (tissue covering the brain and spinal cord) that is usually not cancer. *See also* Brain Tumor (pages 157–159).

**menogaril** Also known by the trade name Menogarol®, this drug belongs to a group of drugs known as anthracycline antibiotics. It is being studied in the treatment of several types of cancer.

**Menogarol®** *See* Menogaril.

**menopause** Permanent cessation of menstruation, or change of life, which in females in the United States usually occurs between 45 and 50 years of age. A woman, regardless of her age, is considered post-menopausal if she has not had a menstrual period for 12 consecutive months. Menopause at an early age, either natural or following the removal of both ovaries, reduces the risk of breast cancer unless replacement estrogen is taken. Conversely, delayed menopause increases the risk of breast malignancy.

**meperidine hydrochloride** Also known by the trade name Demerol®, this is a synthetic opioid similar to morphine. It is used to relieve moderate to severe acute pain, such as after surgery, rather than for the management of chronic cancer pain.

**mercaptopurine** Also known as 6-MP and by the trade name Purinethol®, this drug belongs to a group of drugs known as antimetabolites. It is used to treat several types of cancer, including leukemia.

**Merkel cell carcinoma** A rare, very aggressive skin cancer, which occurs most often in older white people around the head and neck areas exposed to the sun. It presents as a painless, round, shiny, reddish-blue, rapidly growing skin growth. Spread to both lymph nodes and internal organs occurs early. Treatment includes surgical removal of the lesion and margin of normal skin, and adjacent (regional) lymph nodes. In addition to surgery, radiation therapy and chemotherapy may be advised. *See also* Skin Cancer (pages 199–201).

℞ **mesna** Also known by the trade name Mesnex®, this drug is used to prevent hemorrhagic cystitis (severe bladder irritation with bleeding) caused by the chemotherapy agent ifosfamide (Ifex®).

℞ **Mesnex®** *See* Mesna.

**mesothelium** *See* Mesothelioma (pages 184–185).

**metabolism** The sum of all chemical and physical processes in a living organism that is responsible for energy, and tissue growth and repair.

℞ **Metamucil®** *See* Psyllium Hydrophilic Muciloid.

**metastasis** The spread of disease to different sites in the body; often used to describe the appearance of cancer remote from the original or primary location. Metastasis occurs from malignant cells disseminated through lymphatics and blood or by direct extension (seeding) in body spaces such as abdomen, brain, and spinal cord (central nervous system or CNS). Usual sites for metastasis include the lymph nodes, lung, liver, brain, and bone. Metastasis is the usual cause of death in most cancers other than brain tumors.

**metastasize** To spread by metastasis, most often used to describe the dissemination of cancer.

℞ **methadone** Also known by the trade names Dolophine® and Methadose®, this drug belongs to a group of drugs known as synthetic opioid analgesics. It is similar to morphine, and is frequently used to treat patients addicted to heroin. It is also effective in the treatment of moderate to severe pain.

℞ **Methadose®** *See* Methadone.

℞ **methotrexate** Also known by the trade names Amethopterin®, Mexate®, and Folex®, this antimetabolite type of chemotherapy drug was developed more than 40 years ago. It is used to treat many different cancers including breast, head and neck, and bone as well as some types of leukemia. It can be given by mouth, vein, artery, and injected into spinal fluid. The main side effects are suppression of bone marrow and mucositis (severe irritation of the lining of the mouth and throat).

℞ **methyl-CCNU** Also known by the trade names Semustine® and MeCCNU®, this drug belongs to a group of drugs known as alkylating agents. It is a nitrosourea that crosses the blood-brain barrier, and is used to treat several types of cancer, including some brain cancers.

℞ **methylcellulose** Also known by the trade name Citrucel®, this drug is a bulk-producing laxative used to treat constipation.

℞ **metoclopramide** Also known by the trade name Reglan®, this oral and injectable drug is used to control nausea. It appears to work by counteracting the effect of the hormone dopamine on the brain.

℞ **metronizadole hydrochloride** Also known by the trade name Flagyl®, this drug belongs to a general group of drugs known as antibiotics. An unusual side effect of this antibiotic is a potentially severe reaction if patients taking this medication also consume alcohol.

℞ **Mexate®** *See* Methotrexate.

℞ **Mezlin®** *See* Mezlocillin Sodium.

℞ **mezlocillin sodium** Also known by the trade name Mezlin®, this drug is an antibiotic that belongs to a general group of drugs known as penicillins.

℞ **miconazole nitrate** Also known by the trade name Monistat®, this drug is an antifungal agent.

**microcalcifications** *See* Calcifications.

**microscope** A device for magnifying minute objects. The light microscope uses visible light to identify cancer cells and diagnose malignant disease. The electron microscope uses electron beams to achieve greater magnification and is valuable in cancer research. An operating microscope is used to magnify a surgeon's vision during operations on the brain, eye, blood vessels, etc.

**Miles' resection** *See* Abdominoperineal Resection.

℞ **Minocin®** *See* Minocycline Hydrochloride.

℞ **minocycline hydrochloride** Also known by the trade names Minocin®, Vectrin®, and Dynacin®, this is a tetracycline antibiotic active against bacteria and organisms known as *Mycobacterium* and *Chlamydia*.

℞ **Mithracin®** *See* Plicamycin.

℞ **mitomycin** Also known by the trade name Mitomycin C®, this is an anticancer antibiotic used in the treatment of pancreatic cancer and other malignancies of the gastrointestinal (GI) tract as well as breast, lung, cervix, and bladder cancers. Nausea, vomiting, and malaise (feeling poorly) are common unwanted side effects. Mitomycin that leaks from a vein can cause severe chemical injury of the skin and of the fatty subcutaneous tissue beneath the skin that may require a skin graft.

℞ **mitoxantrone** Also known by the trade name Novantrone®, this is an antibiotic drug used in the treatment of several types of cancer, including leukemia.

**modified radical mastectomy** Amputation of the breast that preserves the large muscle underneath the breast (pectoralis major), which is removed in radical mastectomy. Today, this operation is used only for treatment of breast cancer that cannot be removed adequately by lumpectomy or other breast-conserving operations. *See also* Mastectomy.

**modified radical neck dissection** Surgical removal of the lymph nodes on one or both sides of the neck, which preserves the muscles and nerves that are removed in radical neck dissection. The surgery is used for treating head and neck cancers, thyroid cancers, and melanoma and skin cancer of the face and scalp.

**Mohs' surgery** An operation to remove basal cell and squamous cell skin cancers in which successive small amounts of tumor are removed and examined by frozen section until no more cancer is encountered. The operation causes little scarring, but is quite labor-intensive and time-consuming. *See also* Skin Cancer (pages 199–201).

℞ **Monistat®** *See* Miconazole Nitrate.

**monoclonal antibody** An antibody produced by a single cell or its offspring, which is specific for a given antigen. Certain ones are used to diagnose cancers difficult to identify by usual means, and others are being studied intensively as cancer immunotherapy. Rituximab (Rituxan®), a monoclonal antibody, is used as immunotherapy for low-grade B cell lymphoma that persists or recurs after chemotherapy. Another antibody, called alemtuzumab (Campath®), has more recently been approved for the treatment of patients with advanced chronic lymphocytic leukemia.

**morbidity** A measure of the new cases of a disease in a population; the number of people who have a disease; an index of the severity of a medical illness or surgical procedure.

℞ **morphine** Also known by the trade names Astramorph®, Duramorph®, Oramorph®, Roxanol®, and MS Contin®, this opioid is the most widely used drug for pain control. It is very effective, relatively cheap, and can be given by mouth, injection, or rectal suppository. The main drawbacks or side effects are drowsiness and constipation. When used to relieve pain, morphine is unlikely to cause drug addiction.

**mortality** A measure of the rate of death from a disease within a given population.

**6-MP** *See* Mercaptopurine.

**MRI** *See* Magnetic Resonance Imaging.

**MS Contin®** *See* Morphine.

**mucosa** The velvety, inner lining of tube-like organs or portion of organs. It is made up of a layer of cells (epithelium) with an underlying layer of stronger connective tissue. Mucosa is the site of many malignant tumors (non-small cell lung, colorectal, stomach, head-neck, and bladder cancers).

**mucositis** Irritation of the mucosa (lining) of the tongue, mouth, and throat that can cause painful ulcers; most often caused by chemotherapy, such as methotrexate, and by radiation therapy to the head and neck. Although mucositis is usually temporary, it can interfere with eating and cause severe nutritional problems. Treatment consists of mouthwash, and rinses with local anesthetics that numb the mouth.

**mucus** The thick fluid secreted by mucous membranes and glands.

**multidrug resistance** Resistance of a tumor cell to several unrelated drugs after exposure to a single chemotherapy drug.

**multiple endocrine neoplasia (MEN)** Any one of three uncommon conditions in which endocrine tumors involve one or more of these glands: pancreas, pituitary, adrenal, parathyroid, and thyroid.

*MEN 1:* Also known as Wermer's syndrome, an inherited condition with hyperparathyroidism (increased activity of the parathyroid glands); hypercalcemia (increased blood calcium); and pancreatic tumors, insulinoma, gastrinoma, glucagonoma that may be malignant.

*MEN 2A:* Also called Sipple's syndrome, an inherited condition that includes hyperparathyroidism, pheochromocytoma, and medullary thyroid cancer.

*MEN 2B:* A condition that may be inherited, which is similar to type MEN 2A, but more aggressive and likely to cause death before age 30 years. Patients characteristically have puffy lips, irregular teeth, and a prominent jaw.

**multiple intestinal polyposis** *See* Familial Adenomatous Polyposis.

**multiple myeloma** *See* Myeloma (pages 185–186).

**muscle** Body tissue capable of movement. It includes skeletal or striated muscle attached to the skeleton, which is under conscious or voluntary control; and smooth muscle, which is present in blood vessels, gastrointestinal tract, skin, eye, and other organs and is not under conscious or voluntary control. Cancer derived from striated muscle is rhabdomyosarcoma, and from smooth muscle is leiomyosarcoma.

℞ **Mustargen®** *See* Mechlorethamine Hydrochloride.

℞ **Mutamycin®** *See* Mitomycin.

**mutation** A change in a gene.

**MYCN** *See* N-myc.

**mycosis fungoides** A rare, slow growing variety of skin lymphoma; a malignancy of T cells, which seldom affects lymph nodes or internal organs until late in the disease. It is distinguished by the appearance of large, firm, reddish tumors that cause painful skin ulcers. Treatment includes chemotherapy, radiation therapy, and ultraviolet therapy (PUVA).

℞ **Mycostatin®** *See* Nystatin.

**myelosuppression** Inhibition of cells produced in bone marrow that causes reduced numbers of certain white blood cells (granulocytopenia), red blood cells (anemia), and platelets (thrombocytopenia), which if severe, can lead to infection, weakness, and bleeding, respectively. This potentially serious (and sometimes fatal) condition in cancer patients is most often due to chemotherapy and less often to radiation therapy and immunotherapy. Leukemia and myeloma involving bone marrow, infection, and malnutrition also cause myelosuppression.

℞ **Myleran®** *See* Busulfan.

# N

**nadir sepsis** Severe infection due to very low numbers of granulocytes (white blood cells in blood that protect against infection). In people with cancer, it is caused most often by the adverse effects of chemotherapy on bone marrow, where granulocytes are formed. Nadir sepsis may cause only fever and may not cause the usual signs and symptoms of localized infection (pain, tenderness, warmth), which often makes it difficult to diagnose.

**nafcillin sodium** Also known by the trade name Unipen®, this drug is an antibiotic that belongs to a general group of drugs known as semi-synthetic penicillins.

**nasal** Referring to the nose.

**nasal cancer** *See* Head and Neck Cancer (pages 170–172).

**natural killer (NK) cell** A type of white blood cell that is neither of B cell nor T cell origin. It is able to destroy malignant cells grown artificially in tissue culture in the laboratory. Natural killer cells, unlike lymphokine-activated killer (LAK) cells, do not require activation by the cytokine interleukin-2 (IL-2) to destroy cancer cells. Today, both NK and LAK cells are being studied extensively as cancer immunotherapy. *See also* Immunotherapy.

**nausea** A feeling of sickness accompanied by a loathing for food and a desire to vomit or throw up (emesis); a common and one of the most severe side effects of chemotherapy and less often, radiation therapy and immunotherapy. It can also be associated with pain medication, especially morphine, and is a common symptom of increased pressure in the skull as occurs in brain tumors. When associated with vomiting, it can lead to rapid dehydration and chemical (electrolyte) imbalance. Antiemetic drugs given before cancer therapy in most cases make nausea much less severe and treatment more tolerable.

**Navelbine®** *See* Vinorelbine.

**Nebcin®** *See* Tobramycin Sulfate.

**neck dissection** Lymphadenectomy (surgical removal of lymph nodes) in the side of the neck and under the chin. It is used in treating cancers of the head and neck, larynx, and thyroid, as well as melanomas and skin cancers of the face and scalp. Whether or not all of the cervical (neck) nodes, even those not enlarged and unlikely to contain metastatic cancer, need to be removed in every case is controversial. In the past, radical neck dissection, which also removes the large muscle (sternocleidomastoid) in the side of the neck, spinal accessory nerve that lifts the shoulder, and large jugular vein was considered the operation of choice. Today, in selected cases, modified radical and selective neck dissections, both of which preserve the large muscle, major nerves, and large vein, can give similar results without the many problems associated with the disfiguring radical operation.

**needle aspiration** A type of needle biopsy. The removal of fluid from a cyst or cells from a tumor. In this procedure, a needle is used to reach the cyst or tumor, and with suction, aspirate (draw up) samples for examination under the microscope.

**needle biopsy** *See* Biopsy.

**needle localization** A procedure used to guide a surgical breast biopsy when the lump is hard to locate or when there are areas that look suspicious on the x-ray but there is not a distinct lump. A thin needle is placed into the breast and x-rays are taken and used to guide the needle to the suspicious area.

℞ **nefazodone hydrochloride** Also known by the trade name Serzone®, this drug belongs to a group of drugs known as antidepressants.

**neoadjuvant therapy** Cancer treatment, most often chemotherapy, given prior to surgery to shrink a large cancer or tumor, such as inflammatory breast cancer, and make it more manageable. *See also* Adjuvant Therapy.

**neoplasm** Any abnormal tissue that grows more rapidly than normal tissue and forms a mass or lump. A neoplasm may be either benign (noncancerous) or malignant (cancerous), but the term is most often used to mean cancer. *See also* Malignancy; Tumor.

**nephrectomy** Surgical removal of the kidney. A radical nephrectomy that removes both the adjacent adrenal gland and Gerota's fascia (thick tissue surrounding the kidney) remains the standard treatment for cancer limited to the kidney. The operation is done either through the abdomen or side, depending upon tumor size and patient build. More recently, there has been interest in removing cancerous kidneys by laparoscopy, a time consuming but less invasive procedure. *See also* Kidney Cancer (pages 173–174); Laparoscopy.

**nephroblastoma** *See* Wilms' Tumor (pages 212–213).

℞ **Neumega®** *See* Oprelvekin.

℞ **Neupogen®** *See* Filgrastim.

**neurilemoma** A nonmalignant brain tumor that most often involves the nerve to the ear (auditory or cranial nerve VIII). It arises in Schwann cells that form the sheath (nerve covering). Also called cerebellopontine angle tumor; acoustic schwannoma; acoustic neuroma.

**neuroendocrine tumor** Any one of a variety of uncommon, hormone-producing tumors, which includes carcinoid, pheochromocytoma, and paraganglioma. Also called glomus tumor. *See* Carotid Body Tumor.

**neurofibroma** A firm, benign (noncancerous) tumor originating in Schwann cells that form the covering or sheath around nerves outside the central nervous system (brain and spinal cord).

**neurofibromatosis** Either one of two inherited disorders that feature neurofibroma (nerve tumors) and brown (cafe-au-lait) skin spots. Type 1 (NF1) includes cafe-au-lait spots, skin neurofibromas, and benign tumor (hamartoma) of the iris called Lisch nodules. In addition, malignancies such as neurofibrosarcoma, malignant pheochromocytoma, and leukemia may be present. Type 2 (NF2), which is similar to but more rare than NF1, includes vestibular schwannoma (benign tumor of the nerve to the ear) as well as neurofibromas and spots of the skin. In some cases, neurofibromas form large skin lumps that may be very disfiguring.

**neurofibrosarcoma** A cancer affecting nerves outside the central nervous system (brain and spinal cord); the malignant form of neurofibroma. The tumor occurs most often in nerves next to the spine and mediastinum (middle of the chest), and are usually larger than 2 inches in diameter. This type of soft tissue cancer tends to involve adjacent tissue, metastasize early, and often recurs after treatment. *See also* Sarcoma; Soft Tissue Cancer (pages 202–204).

℞ **Neurontin®** *See* Gabapentin.

**neuropathy** *See* Peripheral Neuropathy.

**neurovascular bundle** One of two groups of nerves and blood vessels that run alongside the prostate and help the penis become erect. Removal of or injury to these bundles during surgery, or damage from radiation therapy, can lead to impotence.

℞ **Neutrexin®** *See* Trimetrexate.

**neutron therapy** A type of radiation therapy to treat cancer, which uses high-energy, electrically neutral particles (neutrons) present in the nucleus (at the center) of most atoms. It has proven especially useful in treating salivary gland tumors, melanomas, and soft tissue sarcomas, as well as advanced prostate and head and neck cancers.

**neutropenia** A decrease in the number of neutrophils (white blood cells also known as granulocytes) concerned primarily with protecting the body against infection from bacteria and fungi. *See also* Granulocyte.

**neutrophil** Also called polymorphonuclear leukocyte. *See* Granulocyte.

**nevus** A benign mole or birthmark, which can give rise to superficial spreading melanoma. Those likely to undergo malignant change include a bathing suit nevus, which covers a large area of the body, and a dysplastic nevus (a dark lesion with an irregular outline), which is difficult to distinguish from melanoma without a biopsy. Even without a family history of melanoma, people with large numbers of small nevi appear at greater risk for melanoma. Any mole that attracts attention (itching, bleeding, change in color, size, or shape) should be evaluated immediately by a physician.

℞ **Nilandron®** *See* Nilutamide.

℞ **nilutamide** Also known by the trade name Nilandron®, it belongs to a group of drugs known as hormone antagonists, which block the effect of a hormone. Used to treat advanced prostate cancer, it stops the growth of cancer cells that depend on the male hormone testosterone to grow and divide.

℞ **Nipent®** *See* Pentostatin.

**nipple discharge** Any fluid coming from the nipples that may be clear, milky, bloody, tan, gray, or green.

℞ **nitrogen mustard** *See* Mechlorethamine Hydrochloride.

**nitroimidazole** A chemical compound that makes hypoxic cells (cells with a low oxygen content) more sensitive to the effects of radiation. The presence of hypoxic cancer cells is thought responsible for the failure of some malignant tumors to respond to radiation therapy. *See also* Hyperoxygenation; Hypoxic Cell Sensitizer.

℞ **nitrosourea** Any one of several cancer chemotherapy drugs, such as carmustine (BCNU® and BiCNU®), lomustine (CCNU®), and methyl-CCNU (MeCCNU®) that act similarly to alkylating types of anticancer drugs. Unlike other chemotherapy agents, nitrosoureas are able to penetrate brain tissue through the blood (blood-brain barrier), which makes them useful for treating brain tumors.

℞ **Nizoral®** *See* Ketoconazole.

**NMP22** A protein found in cells lining the bladder, which is increased in bladder cancer. It is the basis for a new urine test that helps individualize treatment by identifying people at increased (or decreased) risk for recurrent bladder cancer who need more (or less) aggressive treatment.

**NMR** Nuclear magnetic resonance imaging, the original name for the imaging technique MRI. The term is no longer used because of dissatisfaction with the term nuclear. *See* MRI.

**N-myc** An oncogene identified with advanced stages of the childhood cancer, neuroblastoma; the result of a chromosome abnormality having additional genes (gene amplification). Also called MYCN. *See* Neuroblastoma (pages 187–188).

**nocturia** Frequent nighttime urination.

**nodal status** Indicates whether a cancer has spread (node-positive) or has not spread (node-negative) to lymph nodes.

**nodular melanoma** *See* Melanoma (pages 182–184).

℞ **Nolvadex®** *See* Tamoxifen.

**nonseminoma** A variety of testicular cancer that accounts for almost 50% of malignant tumors of the testes. Subtypes include embryonal carcinoma, choriocarcinoma, yolk sac tumor, and malignant teratoma.

**non-small cell lung cancer (NSLC)** The most common variety of lung cancer. It includes squamous cell carcinoma, adenocarcinoma, and large cell (undifferentiated) carcinoma. *See also* Lung Cancer (pages 180–182).

**norepinephrine** A hormone similar to epinephrine (adrenaline), both of which are produced in the medulla or central part of the adrenal gland, but having a greater effect than epinephrine in increasing blood pressure. Excessive amounts of both hormones are produced by the adrenal tumor known as pheochromocytoma. *See also* Epinephrine.

℞ **Norpramin®** *See* Desipramine Hydrochloride.

℞ **nortriptyline hydrochloride** Also known by the trade names Aventyl® and Pamelor®, this drug belongs to a group of drugs known as tricyclic antidepressants.

℞ **Novantrone®** *See* Mitoxantrone.

**nutrition** *See* Dietary Fat.

℞ **nystatin** Also known by the trade name Mycostatin®, this is an antifungal antibiotic used to treat fungus infections of the skin and mouth (thrush), the latter is often associated with mucositis (severe oral irritation) from cancer chemotherapy. It is given usually as a liquid swished in the mouth for several minutes and then swallowed. Nystatin ointment and powder are used for skin infections.

# O

**oat cell carcinoma** A variety of small cell lung cancer (SCLC). *See also* Lung Cancer (pages 182–184); Small Cell Carcinoma.

**obesity** The condition of being excessively overweight, which puts women at increased risk for cancers of the uterus (endometrium). Obesity is also associated with an increased risk of colon cancer and, in postmenopausal women, breast cancer. *See also* Dietary Fat.

**occult primary cancer** A cancer that comes from an unidentified site or organ, that makes its presence known by metastases to lymph node(s) or other sites. *See* Primary Cancer.

℞ **octreotide** Also known by the trade name Sandostatin®, this drug is used to treat the symptoms of carcinoid and other hormone-producing tumors, including VIPoma. Its actions are similar to somatostatin, a natural hormone that inhibits the release of other hormones including serotonin and gastrin.

**ocular melanoma** *See* Uveal Melanoma.

**oligodendroglioma** A relatively rare, often slow growing brain tumor of adults that arises in glial cells, which along with neurons or nerves cells make up brain and spinal cord tissue. *See also* Brain Tumor (pages 157–159).

**omentectomy** Surgical removal of the omentum, the fatty apron in the abdomen that is commonly the site of tumor spread from ovarian cancer.

℞ **Omnicef®** *See* Cefdinir.

**oncogene** A damaged version of a type of gene (proto-oncogene) that regulates many vital processes in the body, including cell growth. Oncogenes appear to cause cancer by altering chromosomes. Although different viruses are known to be the source of oncogenes in cats, chickens, rats, and mice, this has not been shown in humans.

**oncologist** A physician who specializes in treating cancer. Included in this group who receive special training are medical oncologists who treat cancer with chemotherapy and immunotherapy, radiation oncologists who treat malignancy with x-rays and other radiation, and surgical oncologists who operate to biopsy, stage, and control malignant tumors.

℞ **Oncovin®** *See* Vincristine.

℞ **ondansetron** Also known by the trade name Zofran®, this drug is given intravenously or orally for nausea and vomiting control and is especially useful in cancer patients who are given chemotherapy, notably cisplatin. It appears to act by interfering with the hormone serotonin.

℞ **Ontak®** *See* Denileukin Diftitox.

**oophorectomy** Surgical removal of one or both ovaries (castration). It is used in ovarian and other female cancers to remove tumors and in breast cancer to eliminate the primary source of the female hormone estrogen. *See also* Breast Cancer (pages 159–161); Ovarian Cancer (pages 190–191).

℞ **opioid** A narcotic drug used alone or with nonopioid drugs (acetaminophen, aspirin) to treat moderate to severe pain. Opioids are similar to natural substances (endorphins) produced by the body to control pain. Some work better than others in relieving severe pain. These medicines were once made from the opium poppy, but today many are synthetic, that is, they are chemicals made by drug companies.

℞ **oprelvekin** Also known by the trade name Neumega®, this hormone-like protein (cytokine) directly stimulates the growth of stem cells, which results in increased platelet production. It is used to prevent thrombocytopenia (a severe reduction in the number of platelets) and the risk of bleeding in patients receiving chemotherapy. Its main adverse effect is fluid retention.

**oral** Relating to the mouth.

**oral cancer** *See* Head and Neck Cancer (pages 170–172).

℞ **Oramorph®** *See* Morphine.

**orchiectomy** Surgical removal of one or both testicles or testes, which are the primary source of the male hormone testosterone. Removal of one testis is used to treat testicular cancer, and removal of both (bilateral orchiectomy or castration) is used to reduce the level of testosterone in the treatment of advanced stage prostate and male breast cancers. *See also* Breast Cancer (pages 159–161); Prostate Cancer (pages 194–196); Testicular Cancer (pages 206–207).

**organ** Any body part having a specific function or purpose (digestion, elimination, reproduction, locomotion).

**osteoarthropathy** Expansion of the ends of bones; a paraneoplastic (associated with cancer) syndrome that causes bone and joint pain. Swelling of the finger tips may be noticed in both non-small cell lung cancer (NSCLC) and chronic lung disease such as emphysema. *See also* Non-Small Cell Lung Cancer; Paraneoplastic Syndrome.

**osteogenic sarcoma** *See* Osteosarcoma.

**osteosarcoma** The most common and potentially dangerous primary bone cancer, which involves bone-forming cells and occurs most often around the knee joint and the upper arm at the shoulder. It is a malignant tumor primarily of children and young adults between the ages of 10 and 25. Before the 1980s, treatment was usually amputation, but today, chemotherapy in addition to surgery enables limb-sparing operations that remove only the tumor and adjacent bone to give as good results. Surgical removal of pulmonary metastasis (cancer spread to the lung) cures some patients. Also called osteogenic sarcoma. *See also* Bone Cancer (pages 156–157).

**ostomy** A surgically created passage between two organs, which may be temporary or permanent. It is often used to describe an opening between the skin and an internal organ, such as in the stomach (gastrostomy), colon (colostomy), or ileum (ileostomy). Also called stoma.

**outpatient** A patient who does not have to stay overnight in the hospital while receiving medical or surgical treatment.

**ovary** The ovaries are a pair of small, female organs in the pelvic area. They are the main source of estrogen, and in the nonpregnant state, progesterone. *See* Ovarian Cancer (pages 190–191).

℞ **oxacillin sodium** Also known by the trade names Bactocill® and Prostaphlin®, this drug is an antibiotic that belongs to a general group of drugs known as semisynthetic penicillins. It is commonly used to treat infections with staphylococci bacteria.

℞ **oxaliplatin** This investigational drug belongs to a group of drugs known as alkylating agents, and specifically is a member of the platinum family of chemotherapy drugs. It is being tested as a treatment for several types of cancer, including colon, breast, and ovarian cancer.

℞ **oxazepam** Also known by the trade name Serax®, this is an anxiolytic (anxiety reliever) drug that belongs to a group of drugs known as benzodiazepines.

℞ **oxycodone** Also known by the trade names Percodan®, Percocet®, and Endodan®, this drug is a synthetic opioid analgesic used as a pain reliever. It is similar to morphine.

# P

**P53** One of the tumor suppressor genes, which when mutated can influence a wide spectrum of tumors. Changes of these and similar genes may also be responsible for making some cancers more likely to grow and spread more rapidly than others.

℞ **paclitaxel** Also known by the trade name Taxol®, this is one of the most widely used chemotherapy drugs. It is particularly useful in controlling advanced ovarian and breast cancers. The most significant adverse effects is neutropenia or marked decrease in the number of neutrophils (a type of white blood cell), which can lead to severe bacterial infections.

**Paget's disease** Three distinct diseases having nothing in common but their name. Paget's disease of the breast is an uncommon breast cancer that causes burning, itching, bleeding, and oozing of the nipple due to a tumor beneath the nipple, which may be either ductal carcinoma in situ (DCIS) or more advanced cancer. It is diagnosed by finding unusual cancer cells (Paget cells) upon biopsy of the nipple. In more than half the cases, a breast lump can be felt or seen on mammograms. As with other more common breast malignancies, the outlook is related to the stage of the underlying cancer. The usual treatment is total mastectomy (removal of the breast), but in some cases, removal of the nipple and central part of the breast may be considered.

Extramammary Paget's disease is a rare skin cancer of the genitals or area around the anus in both men and women. Treatment removes the tumor with a margin of surrounding normal skin.

Paget's disease of bone is a benign (noncancerous) disease of older people that causes thickening and softening of the skull and bones in the legs, which can lead to osteosarcoma (bone cancer) in 1% of cases. *See also* Breast Cancer (pages 159–161); Mastectomy; Osteosarcoma; Skin Cancer (pages 199–201).

**pain** An unpleasant sensation that varies from mild to excruciating; a prominent persistent symptom of advanced or recurrent malignant disease and an initial and usually temporary side effect of cancer treatment. The pain of advanced malignancies is best controlled by therapy directed at the cancer. However, in cases of pain caused from advanced disease, discomfort is usually controlled and made tolerable using narcotics combined with antianxiety drugs. Persons receiving narcotics for chronic pain are unlikely to become addicted and to suffer withdrawal symptoms (the physical and mental disturbances that occur when a drug abuser is denied narcotics) when narcotic medication is gradually reduced as discomfort subsides. It is important to remember that pain may go untreated in the very young and old because they may have difficulty communicating their discomfort.

**palliate** To reduce the severity of a condition; most often applied to the relief of symptoms, particularly pain.

**palliative therapy** Treatment used to relieve symptoms (usually pain) rather than cure disease. Many people with incurable malignancy who receive palliative therapy can live for extended periods in relative comfort. Because of potential adverse effects, even palliative treatment must be weighed against no treatment to ensure that a person with incurable cancer has the best quality of life. In no instance should palliative therapy cause problems more severe than those related to the cancer.

**palpation** Using the hands to examine. A palpable mass in the breast is one that can be felt.

℞ **Pamelor®** *See* Nortriptyline Hydrochloride.

℞ **pamidronate disodium** Also known by the trade name Aredia®, this drug belongs to a group of drugs known as biphosphonates. It is a calcium-lowering drug, and is used to prevent bone from breaking down. In cancer patients, the drug is used to treat abnormally elevated levels of calcium in the blood.

**Pancoast syndrome** Symptoms caused by cancer at the top of the lung (Pancoast tumor) invading the upper part of the chest and involving nerves to the shoulder and neck. Symptoms include chest, shoulder, and arm pain, hand weakness, and Horner's syndrome. *See also* Lung Cancer (pages 180–182).

**Pancoast tumor** Also called superior pulmonary sulcus tumor. *See* Pancoast Syndrome.

**pancolitis** Ulcerative colitis that involves the entire colon.

**pancreas** The pancreas is an organ concerned with digestion; a soft, spongy tube-like gland that lies in front of the spine behind the retroperitoneum (abdominal cavity). *See also* Head of Pancreas; Pancreatic Cancer (pages 191–193).

**pancreatectomy** Surgery to remove the pancreas. *See also* Pancreatic Cancer (pages 191–193).

**pancreatic** Relating to the pancreas. *See* Pancreatic Cancer (pages 191–193).

℞ **Panmycin®** *See* Tetracycline Hydrochloride.

℞ **Panretin®** *See* Alitretinoin Gel 0.1%.

**Pap smear** *See* Pap Test.

**Pap test** The Papanicolaou (Pap) test uses microscopic examination of cells scraped from the lining of the cervix or vagina. Used especially for detecting cervical cancer, it is accurate, painless, readily available, and inexpensive. The availability of the Pap test has played a large role in reducing the number of deaths of American women from cervical cancer over the last half century. Also called Pap smear. *See* Appendix for Cancer Detection Guidelines; Cervical Cancer (pages 161–163).

**papillary carcinoma** Several unrelated cancers. Most often, a common variety of thyroid cancer, but also an inherited type of kidney cancer; and rarely, an early spreading, eccrine (sweat gland) skin cancer of the finger or toe.

**papilloma** Any small, wart-like, benign (noncancerous) growth that arises in epithelial tissue (skin, lining of organs and glands). Papilloma of the bladder is treated with electrocautery (electric current) using a cystoscope. People with bladder papilloma need regular cystoscopic examinations because they are at increased risk for recurrent tumors elsewhere in their urinary system.

**papillomavirus** *See* Human Papillomavirus.

**paracentesis** Removal of fluid from the abdomen using a needle, or hollow tube (trocar or canula) punctured through the abdominal wall. Large amounts of fluid due to an abdominal malignancy, and often occurring with ovarian cancer, are best controlled by means of a Denver® shunt. *See also* Ascites; Denver® Shunt; LeVeen Shunt.

**paraganglioma** A variety of neuroendocrine tumor. Also called glomus tumor. *See* Carotid Body Tumor.

**paraneoplastic syndrome** Any one of a variety of conditions associated with cancer, but not directly related to the malignancy itself. These problems occur most often from cancers of the lung, liver, and kidney, which produce different hormones and unidentified chemical compounds. The more common conditions are weight loss, fever, anemia, weakness, phlebitis (inflamed veins), clubbing (swollen fingertips), hypercalcemia (increased calcium in blood), and skin problems including blisters, cracking, and color change. Most paraneoplastic syndromes disappear when the underlying cancer is controlled.

 **Paraplatin®** *See* Carboplatin.

**parasite** An animal or plant that lives off or is nourished by another living organism; the cause of many different diseases in humans and animals. Parasitic infections that cause chronic irritation of the bladder and bile duct can lead to cancers in these organs.

**parathormone** The hormone produced by the parathyroid gland that increases the level of calcium in the blood. Also known as parathyroid hormone and PTH.

**parathyroid** One of four small glands adherent to the thyroid gland that produce the hormone parathormone; rarely the site of cancer, but commonly the site of adenomas (benign tumors) that produce excess parathormone and cause hyperparathyroidism. *See* Multiple Endocrine Neoplasia (MEN).

**parathyroid hormone** *See* Parathormone.

 **Paregoric®** *See* Camphorated Opium Tincture.

**parotid cancer** *See* Salivary Gland Cancer (pages 198–199).

**parotid gland** The largest of the salivary glands, one in front of each ear, that produce saliva to moisten the mouth and food, and aid in digesting starch.

℞ **paroxetine hydrochloride** Also known by the trade name Paxil®, this drug belongs to a group of drugs known as antidepressants.

℞ **Pathocil®** *See* Dicloxacillin Sodium.

**pathologist** A physician who examines biopsy material and other tissue for the presence of cancer and other diseases. Pathologists supervise diagnostic laboratories and hospital blood banks and perform autopsies and needle biopsies.

℞ **Paxil®** *See* Paroxetine Hydrochloride.

**PDT** *See* Photodynamic Therapy.

**pelvic examination** An examination of a woman's uterus and other pelvic organs. Physicians visually examine external structures and palpate the internal organs such as the ovaries and cervix.

**pelvic node dissection** Removal of the lymph nodes in the pelvis.

**pelvis** The lower part of the abdominal cavity surrounded by the pelvic bones, sacrum, and coccyx.

**penectomy** Amputation of the penis. *See* Penile Cancer (pages 193–194).

℞ **PenG Potassium®** *See* Pencillin G.

℞ **PenG Sodium®** *See* Penicillin G.

℞ **penicillin G** Also known by the trade names PenG Potassium® and PenG Sodium®, this drug is an antibiotic use to treat bacterial infections.

**penile** Referring to the penis. *See* Penile Cancer (pages 193–194).

**penile implant** Artificial device placed in the penis during surgery to restore erections.

**penis** The penis is the male sex organ that contains the urethra, the small passage through which urine is passed and sperm is ejaculated. *See* Penile Cancer (pages 193–194).

℞ **pentostatin** Also known by the trade name Nipent®, this is an antimetabolite type of chemotherapy drug given intravenously to treat leukemia, particularly the hairy cell variety. Unwanted side effects include nephrotoxicity (kidney injury), bone marrow toxicity, nausea and vomiting, and conjunctivitis (eye irritation).

**Percocet®** *See* Oxycodone.

**Percodan®** *See* Oxycodone.

**peripheral neuropathy** Disturbances of nerve(s) in the hands and feet, such as weakness, pain, numbness, tingling, and trembling; caused by either nerve involvement with cancer, radiation therapy, or chemotherapy. In some cases, it is a paraneoplastic syndrome with no obvious cause. Neuropathy due to cisplatin and vinca alkaloids (vincristine, vinblastine) usually improves after chemotherapy is stopped. Nerve problems related to radiation therapy may not appear until many years following treatment. *See also* Paraneoplastic Syndrome.

**perineal prostatectomy** An operation where the prostate is removed through an incision in the skin between the scrotum and anus. *See also* Prostate Cancer (pages 194–196).

**peritoneal cavity** *See* Abdomen.

**peritoneovenous shunt** A device implanted in the body to treat ascites (recurring fluid in the abdomen) due to cancer. *See also* Ascites; Denver® Shunt; LeVeen Shunt.

**peritoneum** The smooth lining that envelops abdominal and pelvic organs and covers the inner surface of the abdomen and pelvic area. It is made up of mesothelium (a thin layer of cells). Although rarely the site of primary cancer (mesothelioma), the peritoneum is commonly involved with tumor spread from cancer in the abdomen, especially ovarian cancer.

**permanent section** A very thin slice of tissue or a group of cells preserved in formaldehyde or another tissue preservative, embedded in a block of paraffin wax, and mounted on a glass slide for examination under a microscope. Permanent sections require at least 12 hours to process, as opposed to the faster (and less detailed) frozen sections that take less than 15 minutes. Samples embedded in wax blocks for permanent sections can be stored at room temperature and retrieved for study after many years.

**perphenazine** Also known by the trade name Trilafon®, this drug belongs to a group of drugs known as phenothiazines. It is used as a treatment for nausea.

**Pertofrane®** *See* Desipramine Hydrochloride.

**PET** *See* Positron Emission Tomography.

**Peutz-Jeghers syndrome (PJS)** An uncommon inherited condition that includes small dark freckles on the lips and inside the mouth, hamartomas (noncancerous tumors) throughout the stomach and intestines, and rare ovarian tumors in young girls. Although hamartomas are not malignant, cancers of the stomach and small intestine are more common in people with PJS.

**Peyer's patches** Collections of densely packed lymphocytes in the small intestine.

℞ **Pharmorubicin®** *See* Epirubicin Hydrochloride.

℞ **Phenergan®** *See* Promethazine Hydrochloride.

**pheochromocytoma** A rare, hormone-producing tumor of the medulla (central part) of the adrenal gland, and less frequently of the autonomic nerves, which is cancerous in only 10% of cases. It may be inherited as part of multiple endocrine neoplasia (MEN) syndrome, in which it occurs simultaneously in both adrenal glands. Both benign and malignant pheochromocytomas produce increased blood levels of hormones from the adrenal medulla. Excess epinephrine (adrenaline) and norepinephrine cause increased blood pressure and heart rate, uncontrolled shaking, and other symptoms such as violent headaches, nausea, anxiety, chest discomfort, and abdominal pain. Increased amounts of adrenal hormones in urine help determine the diagnosis. Although CT and MRI make the diagnosis of pheochromocytoma much easier, these imaging studies do not indicate whether or not a tumor is malignant. Because it is not possible to tell if a pheochromocytoma is malignant from microscopic examination, the diagnosis of cancer depends upon the presence of spread or metastasis. Usual therapy is surgical removal of the adrenal gland or of the entire mass in the case of autonomic nerve tumor. Both chemotherapy and irradiation are used for metastasis.

℞ **Phenameth®** *See* Promethazine Hydrochloride.

**Philadelphia chromosome** An abnormal rearrangement of chromosomes 9 and 22 present in white blood cells taken from some people with leukemia. This chromosomal abnormality (Ph1) is present in 95% of people with chronic myelogenous leukemia (a leukemia of granulocytes or infection fighting white blood cells) and in some individuals with acute myelocytic leukemia. More recent treatment advances for patients with chronic myelogenous leukemia with the drug Gleevec have resulted in prolonged remissions and possibly cures. *See also* Leukemia (pages 176–178).

**photodynamic therapy (PDT)** Cancer treatment using a photosensitizer (a drug such as hematoporphyrin) that makes cancer cells sensitive to visible light. After the medication is given intravenously, either a strong red light or an argon laser directed at the tumor destroys the sensitized malignant cancer cells. Although PDT is successful in treating skin and eye tumors, and temporarily relieving obstruction from esophageal, lung, and rectal cancers, it is not widely available.

℞ **piperacillin sodium** Also known by the trade name Pipracil®, this drug is an antibiotic that belongs to a general group of drugs known as semi-synthetic penicillins.

℞ **piperacillin sodium combined with tazobactam sodium** Also known by the trade names Zosyn® and Tazocin®, this drug combination is an antibiotic that belongs to the penicillin class of antibiotics.

℞ **Pipracil®** *See* Piperacillin Sodium.

**pituitary** A complex gland at the base of the brain that produces a variety of hormones, including adrenocorticotropic hormone (ACTH) that causes the adrenal cortex to release cortisone and other hormones. Pituitary tumors that cause excess hormone production lead to a variety of problems, including Cushing's disease and gigantism (overgrowth of the body). Problems with vision can result from a pituitary tumor pressing on the optic nerve to the eye. *See also* ACTH; Cushing's Syndrome.

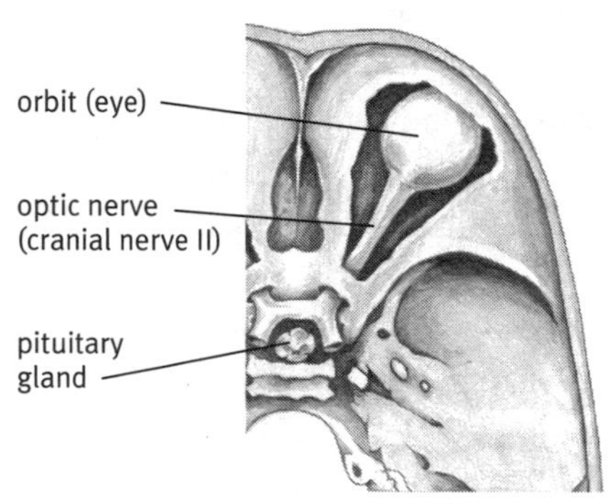

top view of brain

**placebo** An inert, inactive substance that may be used in studies (clinical trials) to compare the effects of a given treatment with no treatment. In common speech, a "sugar pill."

**placenta** The organ in the uterus that connects mother and unborn infant through which oxygen and nutrients are exchanged. It is the site of the rare cancer placental-site trophoblastic tumor. Also called afterbirth.

**plasma** The liquid part of circulating blood that contains antibodies, proteins, and chemical compounds necessary for life.

**platelet** A very small blood cell necessary for coagulation (blood clotting). It is produced in vast numbers in bone marrow from megakaryocytes (much larger cells). Conditions affecting bone marrow, including cytotoxic chemotherapy and bone marrow malignancies (leukemia, myeloma), cause thrombocytopenia (greatly reduced numbers of platelets) that may lead to prolonged bleeding. In addition, leukemia, lymphoma, and other conditions that affect the spleen can cause hypersplenism (where the spleen is markedly enlarged) and result in increased removal of platelets from the blood. Bleeding due to low numbers of platelets is treated with platelet transfusion. Also called thrombocyte.

℞ **Platinol®** *See* Cisplatin.

**pleura** The two layers of mesothelium (very thin filmy tissue), which line the inside of the chest wall (parietal pleura) and cover the lungs (visceral pleura). The potential space between the two pleural layers, which normally are directly adherent to each other, is where fluid (malignant pleural effusion) can accumulate from cancers in the chest. Both the parietal and visceral pleurae are often involved with primary lung cancer, as well as cancer spread from malignancies such as breast cancer. It is much less often the origin of the rare cancer called mesothelioma (cancer arising in pleura). Mesothelioma is commonly associated with exposure to large quantities of asbestos in the workplace. *See also* Mesothelioma (pages 184–185).

**pleural effusion** *See* Effusion.

**pleural mesothelioma** *See* Mesothelioma (pages 184–185).

**pleurectomy** A surgical procedure that strips the lining or pleura from inside the chest, which causes the lungs to adhere to the chest. It is used to obliterate the pleural space between the lungs and prevent malignant pleural effusion (the collection of fluid from cancer in the chest). The surgery is done either by thoracotomy (opening the chest) or endoscopy (thoracoscopy).

℞ **plicamycin** Also known by the trade name Mithracin®, this anticancer antibiotic is used to treat testicular cancer, an accelerated phase of myelogenous leukemia, and to lower hypercalcemia (increased blood calcium) not responsive to usual therapy using large amounts of intravenous fluid and diuretics. Nausea and vomiting are common adverse effects, and almost one-third of treated patients develop epistaxis (severe nosebleed).

**ploidy** Relating to the number of sets of chromosomes in a cell. Except for sex cells (egg and sperm) that are haploid (contain only one chromosomal set), all other human cells are diploid (contain two sets, with each set containing 23 chromosomes). Aneuploidy, the state of having a chromosome number that is not a multiple of the haploid number (abnormal number of chromosome sets), is present in the cells of many different cancers.

**Plummer-Vinson syndrome (PVS)** An uncommon condition with a web-like growth across the upper esophagus that causes difficulty in swallowing. PVS can also include iron deficiency anemia, brittle fingernails, painful irritation of the tongue or glossitis, and splenomegaly (an enlarged spleen). It occurs more often in women, and approximately 10% of affected people develop cancer of the esophagus or throat. *See also* Esophageal Cancer (pages 167–168).

**pneumonectomy** Surgical removal of the lung and adjacent lymph nodes. Once the operation of choice for treating lung cancer, it is now used for non-small cell lung cancer (NSCLC) that cannot be effectively treated by lobectomy (removing only a lobe). Removal of one or two lobes of the lung is much less likely than pneumonectomy to result in pulmonary insufficiency (post-operative breathing difficulty) and heart failure. *See also* Lung Cancer (pages 180–182); Non-Small Cell Lung Cancer.

**pneumonitis** Inflammation in the lung, usually from a bacterial or viral infection. In patients with cancer, irritation of the lung, shortness of breath, persistent cough, and mild chest discomfort can occur as a result of chemotherapy with drugs such as bleomycin or radiation therapy. The problem can progress to scarring of the lung that results in severe permanent breathing difficulty. Depending on the cause, treatment may include antibiotics or cortisone-like medication.

**polymorphonuclear leukocyte** Also called neutrophil. *See* Granulocyte.

**polyp** A piling up of tissue due to either a benign tumor (noncancerous growth) or chronic irritation (inflammation). The growth may be mushroom-shaped with a stalk supporting a rounded tip or head (pedunculated) or sessile (not pedunculated). Adenomatous polyps in the large intestine are thought to be the forerunner of most colorectal cancers and should be removed by colonoscopy to prevent malignancy. Other types of polyps found in the colon, called hyperplastic, are not associated with increased risk of malignancy. The differentiation between types of polyps, and whether or not they already have the early signs of cancer, is made under the microscope. *See also* Colorectal Cancer (pages 163–165).

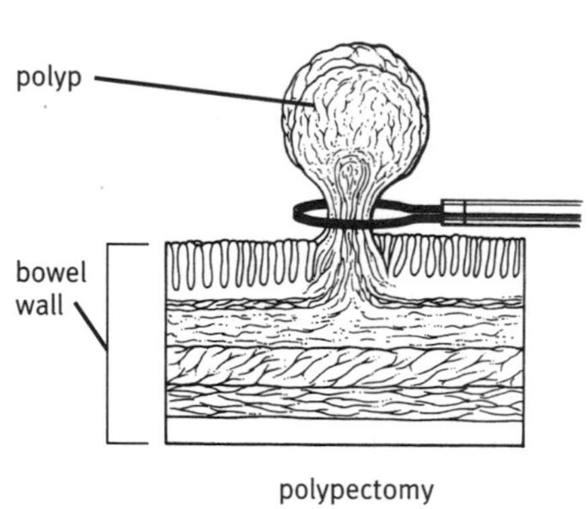

polypectomy

**polypectomy** Surgical removal of a polyp. For colon polyps, polypectomy can usually be done by means of colonoscopy with little discomfort and risk of complications.

**polyposis** *See* Multiple Intestinal Polyposis.

**port** *See* Implantable port.

**portal vein** The large vein that carries blood to the liver from the intestines, stomach, pancreas, and spleen. Malignant cells from cancers in these organs spread via portal venous blood to the liver where they produce secondary cancer (metastasis).

**positive margin** *See* Margin.

**positron emission tomography (PET)** Positron emission tomography is a more recently developed imaging study that shows great promise in detecting and staging cancer. Because the procedure requires a cyclotron (a complex electric device) to produce the necessary, extremely short-lived radioisotopes, the procedure is available only in a few, large cancer treatment centers. *See also* Imaging Study.

**postmenopausal** Relating to the time after menopause (the change of life) when there has not been a menstrual period for the preceding 12 months. Menopause usually occurs between the ages of 45 and 50 in women in the United States. Following bilateral oophorectomy (removal of both ovaries), women who do not receive replacement estrogen are considered to be postmenopasual.

**precancerous** Any lesion from which a cancer is likely to develop (colon polyp, leukoplakia). Also called premalignant.

**predisposition** Susceptibility to a disease that can be triggered under certain conditions. For example, some women have a family history of breast cancer and are therefore more likely to develop breast cancer.

℞ **prednisone** Also known by the trade names Apo-Prednisone® and Deltasone®, this drug is made synthetically and is more potent than the natural hormone cortisol that is produced by the cortex (outer layer) of the adrenal gland. It is used in treating leukemia, Hodgkin's disease, and lymphoma. It is also used to treat hypercalcemia (elevated calcium levels in the blood) associated with these malignancies and other cancer involving bone. *See also* Hodgkin's Disease (pages 172–173); Leukemia (pages 176–178); Non-Hodgkin's Lymphoma (pages 188–190).

**preinvasive cancer** The earliest stage of a malignant tumor, before it invades or grows deeper into underlying tissue. This superficial cancer is cured either by minor surgical removal, electrocautery (electric current), cryotherapy (freezing), or laser. Left untreated, preinvasive cancers can progress to invasive cancer that requires more extensive treatment. *See also* Carcinoma In Situ.

**premalignant** *See* Precancerous.

**premenopausal** Relating to the time before menopause or change of life. A woman is considered premenopausal if there has not been a single menstrual period in the preceding 12 months.

**preoperative** Relating to the time immediately prior to a surgical procedure (operation).

**prevalence** A measure of the proportion of people in the population with a particular disease at a given time.

**prevention** The reducing of cancer risk by eliminating or reducing contact with cancer causing agents. A change in lifestyle, such as quitting smoking, reduces the risk of many cancers.

**primary cancer** The original or first malignant tumor, which may be the source of metastasis (spread) to lymph nodes and other organs, especially liver, lung, and bone. *See* Occult Primary Cancer.

℞ **Primaxin®** *See* Imipenem/Cilastatin Sodium.

℞ **Prinomastat®** *See* AG3340.

℞ **procarbazine hydrochloride** Also known by the trade name Matulane®, this is a miscellaneous drug (a hydrazine derivative) used in the treatment of several types of cancer, including Hodgkin's disease.

℞ **prochlorperazine** Also known by the trade name Compazine®, this drug has long been used to control nausea. It can be given by mouth, injection, or rectal suppository, and its main undesirable side effect is drowsiness.

℞ **Procrit®** *See* Epoetin.

**proctoscope** *See* Sigmoidoscope.

**proctoscopy** *See* Sigmoidoscopy.

**progesterone** A female hormone produced by the ovaries and placenta (after-birth) during pregnancy. Megestrol (Megace®), an oral synthetic hormone similar to progesterone, is used for treating endometrial and breast cancers and for improving poor appetite (anorexia).

**progesterone receptor assay** A laboratory test done on a piece of the breast cancer tissue that shows whether the cancer depends on progesterone for growth. Progesterone and estrogen receptor tests provide more complete information to help determine the best cancer treatment.

**prognosis** A prediction of the course of disease; the outlook for the cure of the patient.

℞ **promethazine hydrochloride** Also known by the trade names Anergan®, Phenameth®, and Phenergan®, this drug belongs to a general group of drugs known as antihistamines. It is also useful as a treatment for nausea and vomiting.

**prophylactic** Action taken to prevent disease (including cancer), such as the removal of both ovaries or both breasts in women at increased risk for developing either breast or ovarian cancer, or the removal of lymph nodes likely to contain melanoma. Prophylactic antibacterial antibiotics are used to prevent infection. The opposite of therapeutic, in which an action is advised only after a disease, cancer, or infection is present.

 **Prostaphlin®** *See* Oxacillin Sodium.

**prostascint scan** Like the bone scan, the prostascint scan uses low-level radioactive material to find cancer that has spread beyond the prostate. The radioactive material is attached to a monoclonal antibody.

**prostate** The prostate is the walnut-size gland at the base of the bladder; part of the male reproductive system that produces semen, the thick fluid in which sperm are ejaculated. *See also* Prostate Cancer (pages 194–196).

**prostatectomy** Surgical removal of all or part of the prostate, which is done either through the abdomen or perineum (the area between the legs behind the penis and in front of the anus). A radical prostatectomy is surgery to remove the entire prostate gland, seminal vesicles, and nearby tissue. *See also* Prostate Cancer (pages 194–196).

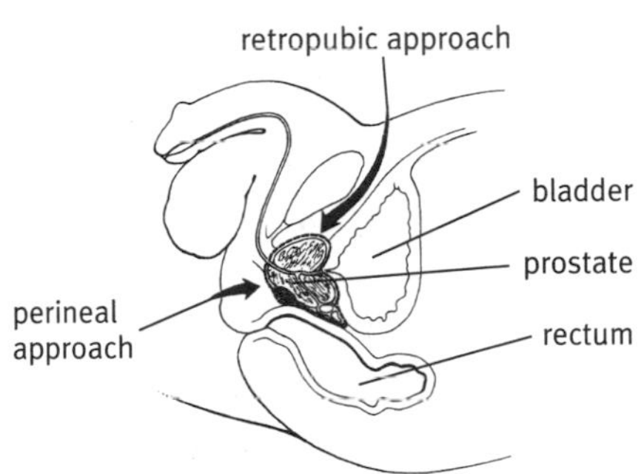


Different approaches to performing radical prostatectomy. Illustration used by permission of Mayo Clinic, ©1996.

**prostate-specific antigen (PSA)** Prostate-specific antigen is a tumor marker in blood used to detect prostate cancer. In those who have been treated for cancer, it is used to indicate a persistent or recurrent tumor that requires additional therapy. PSA may be elevated in the noncancerous condition, benign prostatic hypertrophy (BPH). Sexual activity can raise PSA, and some physicians recommend abstaining from sexual activity for 48 hours before having the blood test. PSA can find prostate cancers early, before they can be detected on physical examination. This offers the best chance for cure before the cancer spreads outside the prostate gland. *See* Appendix for Cancer Detection Guidelines; Prostate Cancer (pages 194–196).

**prostatic intraepithelial neoplasia** A condition in which there are changes in the microscopic appearances of prostate epithelial cells. The condition may lead to the development of prostate cancer. *See also* Prostate Cancer (pages 194–196).

**prostatic urethra** The part of the urethra that runs through the prostate.

**prostatitis** Inflammation of the prostate. Prostatitis is not cancer. It can be acute (sudden) or chronic (long lasting).

**prosthesis** An artificial form, such as a breast prosthesis that may be worn under clothes after a mastectomy.

**protein** Large complex chemical molecules essential for life; present in all cells and in bodily fluids such as blood. All are made up of amino acids, small nitrogen-containing molecules.

℞ **Prozac®** *See* Fluoxetine Hydrochloride.

**PSA** *See* Prostate-Specific Antigen.

**PSA velocity (PSAV)** Measures how quickly the PSA level increases over a period of time. A rapidly rising velocity may be an indicator of cancer in the prostate gland. *See also* Appendix for Cancer Detection Guidelines; Prostate Cancer (pages 194–196); Prostate-Specific Antigen.

**psoralen ultraviolet alpha ray (PUVA)** Therapy to treat mycosis fungoides (skin lymphoma) and skin cancers other than melanoma. Psoralen, a compound that causes skin to become sensitive to ultraviolet radiation, is given by mouth after which the affected area is exposed to ultraviolet alpha (UA) rays. It is also used in the treatment of severe psoriasis, and has been associated with an increased incidence of skin cancers.

℞ **psyllium hydrophilic muciloid** Also known by the trade names Fiberall® and Metamucil®, this is a plant fiber that is used as a bulk-producing laxative.

**PTH** *See* Parathormone.

**pulmonary** Relating to the lungs.

**pulmonary embolism** Complete or partial blockage of one or both pulmonary arteries (large blood vessels) to the lungs caused by an embolus (blood clot) breaking free from a thrombus (larger clot) in a vein in the pelvis or leg. An embolism is a threat to all cancer patients, especially following surgery, and in some cases, may be the first indication of pancreatic cancer. Usual treatment is with anticoagulants (blood-thinning medication). *See also* Embolism.

**pulmonary function test (PFT)** A detailed examination of the lungs that determines their ability to move air in and out, absorb oxygen ($O_2$) from the air, and remove carbon dioxide ($CO_2$) from the blood. In lung cancer patients considered for surgery, PFT is used to determine whether or not they can tolerate pneumonectomy (removal of an entire lung) or lobectomy (removal of only a part of the lung). *See also* Lung Cancer (pages 180–182).

℞ **Purinethol®** *See* Mercaptopurine.

**PUVA** *See* Psoralen Ultraviolet Alpha Ray Therapy.

**pyelogram** An x-ray image obtained by pyelography.

**pyelography** An x-ray study of the kidneys, ureters, and bladder; used to diagnose tumors, stones, and blockage in the urinary tract. Intravenous pyelography (IVP) uses material opaque to x-rays, which is injected into a vein to outline the urinary tract. Retrograde pyelography uses opaque dye placed into the ureter during cystoscopy.

# Q

**quackery** *See* Unproven Treatment.

Rx **Quadramet®** *See* Samarium Sm-153 Lexidronam.

Rx **quinupristin and dalfopristin** Also known by the trade name Synercid®, this drug combination is in the streptogramin class of antibiotics, which is one of the newer classes of antibiotics. It is used to treat bacterial infections that are resistant to other antibiotics, such as vancomycin.

# R

**race** A large population of individuals who display common characteristics. In the United States, there are striking racial differences in the occurrence of different cancers among various racial/ethnic groups. It is not clear how much of this difference is related to common genetic influence and how much is due to similar socioeconomic and environmental conditions.

**RAD** Stands for "radiation absorbed dose," a measurement of the amount of radiation absorbed by tissues.

**radiation proctitis** A possible side effect of external beam radiation therapy. Problems can include pain, bowel frequency, bowel urgency, bleeding, chronic burning, or rectal leakage. *See also* Radiation Therapy.

**radiation therapy** Treatment with high-energy rays (such as x-rays) to kill or shrink cancer cells. The radiation may come from outside of the body (external radiation) or from radioactive materials placed directly in the tumor (internal or implant radiation). Radiation therapy may be used to reduce the size of a cancer before surgery, to destroy any remaining cancer cells after surgery, or, in some cases, as the main treatment. The type of radiation therapy used depends on many factors, including the type of tumor, location, and stage of disease, as well as age, health status, personal preferences, and other factors. *See also* Brachytherapy;

Conformal Proton Beam Irradiation Therapy; External Beam Radiation; Ionizing Radiation; Iridium.

**radical** Any extensive cancer operation formerly deemed always necessary to treat most malignant tumors; includes removal of the cancer, surrounding tissue likely to be involved, and adjacent (regional) lymph nodes. Today, because many tumors are less advanced than in previous years as a result of earlier diagnosis, less extensive surgery (modified radical surgery) combined with drugs and radiation often achieves the same results as more extensive operations, and without many of the adverse effects and risks. *See also* Mastectomy; Prostatectomy.

**radioactive implant** A source of high-dose radiation that is placed directly into or around a tumor to kill the cancer cell. *See also* Brachytherapy; Radiation Therapy.

**radiofrequency interstitial tissue ablation (RITA)** Radiofrequency (RF) uses electrical energy to destroy liver cancers that cannot be removed by surgery. This procedure uses a needle-like electrode through which an electric current is passed into the tumor, destroying it and a small rim of surrounding tissue, both of which are absorbed over time. RITA appears superior to cryotherapy (extreme cold) for treating liver cancer that cannot be removed. *See also* Liver Cancer (pages 178–179).

**radioisotope** Any form of a chemical element, either natural, or more often artificial, which gives off energy in the form of waves or atomic particles. It is used in imaging studies and radiation therapy. *See also* Imaging Study; Radiation Therapy.

**radionuclide bone scan** A study using a small amount of radioisotope to produce images of the bone. It is most frequently used to determine whether or not a cancer has spread (metastasized).

**radium** A naturally radioactive, metallic element extracted from pitchblende ore, which produces x-rays; once widely used in radiation therapy.

**radon** An invisible, odorless, radioactive gas found in rocks and soil, resulting from the breakdown (decay) of radium. It may contribute to a significant number of cases of lung cancer in the United States. Household levels of radon can be measured using commercially available detection kits. Small metal seeds containing radon are used in radiation therapy (brachytherapy) of malignant tumors. *See also* Lung Cancer (pages 180–182).

**Raxar®** *See* Grepafloxacin.

**rectal** Relating to the rectum. *See also* Digital Rectal Exam.

**rectum** Lower part of the large intestine leading to the anus.

**rectum cancer** *See* Colorectal Cancer (pages 163–165).

**recurrence** Cancer that has come back after treatment. Local recurrence means that the cancer has come back at the same site as the original cancer. Regional recurrence means the cancer has come back after treatment in the lymph nodes near the primary site. Distant recurrence is when cancer spreads, after treatment, to other organs or tissues.

**red blood cell (RBC)** A cell that gives blood its distinctive color, whose function is to transport oxygen throughout the body. Upon entering the lungs, blood is exposed to molecular oxygen that binds (attaches) to hemoglobin, a protein-iron compound in red blood cells. As these cells pass through capillaries, the smallest blood vessels that connect arteries and veins, oxygen is released from hemoglobin into surrounding tissue. Similar to platelets and white blood cells, red blood cells are derived from bone marrow stem cells. Also called erythrocyte.

**refractory** No longer responsive to a certain therapy.

**regional enteritis** *See* Crohn's Disease.

**regional node** Any lymph node(s) adjacent to an organ; usually the first site of metastasis (spread) from carcinoma, the most common variety of cancer. Enlarged nodes in the neck, groin, and axilla (underarm) may be the first indication of advanced cancer. Routine lymphadenectomy (removal of regional nodes) adjacent to the tumor has been the usual way to treat most malignant tumors. Today, the sentinel node technique, as used for melanoma and breast cancer, makes it possible to identify regional nodes nearest to the tumor that most likely contain cancer cells (metastasis). This procedure helps determine prognosis and the need for further treatment for patients with melanoma and breast cancer.

**Reglan®** *See* Metoclopramide.

**regression** Reduction of the size of the tumor or the extent of the cancer.

**relapse** Reappearance of cancer after a disease-free period. *See also* Recurrence.

**remission** Complete or partial disappearance of the signs and symptoms of cancer in response to treatment; the period during which a disease is under control. A remission may not be a cure.

**renal** Relating to the kidney.

**renal cell carcinoma** *See* Kidney Cancer (pages 173–174).

**reproductive** Having to do with producing offspring.

**resection** Surgery to remove part or all of an organ or other structure.

**resectoscope** An instrument used in transurethral resection of the prostate (surgical removal of enlarged prostate tissue through the urethra), allowing the surgeon direct inspection of the prostatic urethra and adjacent prostatic tissue.

**respiratory** Having to do with the lungs and breathing.

**retina** The innermost layer of the eye, which converts light into nerve impulses sent to the brain through the optic nerve. *See* Retinoblastoma (pages 196–197).

**retroperitoneal** Referring to the retroperitoneum.

**retroperitoneum** The space behind the abdomen, in front of the back muscles, where the pancreas, kidneys, adrenal glands, lymph nodes, and large blood vessels (aorta and inferior vena cava) are located.

**retropubic** Behind the pubic bone; a surgical approach to the prostate through an incision in the lower abdomen. *See also* Prostatectomy.

**rhabdomyosarcoma** A rare type of muscle cancer; a soft tissue sarcoma that arises in tissues destined to become striated muscle (muscle attached to the skeleton that provides movement). This cancer most often affects children, in whom it can occur in almost any site in the body. Symptoms depend on location, size, and presence of metastases in lymph nodes, lung, and other organs. Treatment that includes surgery, multidrug chemotherapy, and radiation results in curing 64% of cases. *See also* Soft Tissue Cancer (pages 202–204).

**risk factor** Anything that increases a person's chance of getting a disease, such as cancer. Different cancers have different risk factors. Some of these factors, such as smoking, can be changed. Others, like a person's age, cannot.

**RITA** *See* Radiofrequency Interstitial Tissue Ablation.

℞ **Rituxan®** *See* Rituximab.

℞ **rituximab** Also known by the trade name Rituxan®, this is a mouse monoclonal antibody used as immunotherapy for low grade B cell lymphoma that persists or returns following chemotherapy.

℞ **Rocephin®** *See* Ceftriaxone Sodium.

**Roentgen ray** *See* X-ray.

℞ **Roxanol®** *See* Morphine.

**RT-PCR test** The reverse transcriptase-polymerase chain reaction test. A very sensitive test for finding small numbers of cancer cells in blood, bone marrow, and other samples. It is sometimes used to evaluate the success or failure of treatment for some kinds of leukemia because it is able to detect the presence of even a few leukemic cells that would be missed by other tests. It is still uncertain if, or how, the test should be used in considering treatment options for patients with melanoma, prostate cancer, and several other cancers. *See also* Prostate Cancer (pages 194–196).

℞ **Rubidomycin®** *See* Daunorubicin.

# S

**saccharin** The original artificial sweetener found to cause bladder cancer in laboratory animals fed excessive amounts of the compound. However, a large study in humans found little or no increase in bladder cancers in those who consumed beverages and foods containing saccharin. It is unlikely that this sugar substitute taken in usual amounts causes malignant bladder tumors. *See also* Bladder Cancer (pages 154–156).

**salivary gland** The salivary glands are oral glands that produce fluids (saliva) that lubricate the mouth (mucous), soften and dilute food, and convert starch to sugar. *See* Salivary Gland Cancer (pages 198–199).

**salpingo-oophorectomy** Surgical procedure to remove a fallopian tube and adjacent ovary, either unilateral (on one side) or bilateral (both).

℞ **salsalate** Also known by the trade name Disalcid®, this drug belongs to a group of drugs known as nonsteroidal anti-inflammatory drugs (NSAIDs). It is a nonopioid analgesic similar to aspirin, and is used as a pain reliever.

**salvage chemotherapy** *See* Leukemia (pages 176–178).

℞ **samarium Sm-153 lexidronam** Also known by the trade name Quadramet®, this intravenous (IV) medication is used to treat pain caused by cancer spread to bone that causes osteoblastic lesions (new bone growth), often due to advanced prostate, breast, and lung cancers. It consists of the radioactive isotope (samarium-153 [Sm-153]) that delivers radiation, and a compound (lexidronam) that guides the isotope to the new bone growth. The main adverse effect is bone marrow suppression, which lowers the numbers of white blood cells and platelets.

℞ **Sandostatin®** *See* Octreotide.

**sarcoidosis** A disease of unknown origin that can cause enlarged lymph nodes in the chest, which initially is often mistaken for Hodgkin's disease or lymphoma.

**sarcoma** Cancer of connective tissue (tissue made up of similar cells, which surround, connect, bind together, or support organs and body structures). Sarcomas are divided into two major types: soft tissue sarcoma and bone sarcoma, both of which are further divided into several subtypes. Soft tissue sarcoma, the most prevalent type, arises in connective tissue other than bone and includes malignant fibrous histiocytoma (MFH), leiomyosarcoma, liposarcoma, Kaposi's sarcoma, angiosarcoma, neurofibrosarcoma, and rhabdomyosarcoma. Bone sarcoma includes osteosarcoma, chondrosarcoma, and Ewing's sarcoma. Most of these cancers have a tendency to easily spread through the blood, especially to the lung. Treatment varies with the type of tumor, but always includes surgical removal of the primary (original) tumor. *See also* Chondrosarcoma; Ewing's Sarcoma; Kaposi's Sarcoma; Leiomyosarcoma; Liposarcoma; Malignant Fibrous Histiocytoma; Neurofibrosarcoma; Osteosarcoma; Rhabdomyosarcoma; Soft Tissue Cancer (pages 202–204).

℞ **sargramostim** Also known by the trade name Leukine®, this is a cytokine that belongs to the class of artificially synthesized drugs known as biological response modifiers. It is used to prevent fever due to low white blood cell counts following chemotherapy, by increasing the numbers of infection fighting white blood cells and macrophages in the blood.

**SBLA syndrome** *See* Cancer Family Syndrome.

**scan** To survey the body using a sensing device (CT, ultrasound, radioisotope). Also, the image obtained by scanning, often identified by the technique used (MRI, CT scan, ultrasound scan, radioisotope scan). In addition, a term to identify a particular radioisotope scan (brain, liver, or bone scan).

**schwannoma** *See* Neurilemoma.

**scintillation camera** A device used in nuclear medicine scans to detect radioactivity and produce images that help diagnose cancer and other diseases.

**sclerotherapy** Treatment in which a substance that irritates and scars is injected into tissue or blood vessels. *See* Effusion.

℞ **scopolamine** Also known by the trade name Transderm-Scop®, this drug belongs to a group of drugs known as anticholinergics, which block the passage of impulses that stimulate the parasympathetic nerves that control nausea and vomiting. It is frequently used to treat motion sickness.

**screening** The search for disease, such as cancer, in people without symptoms. For example, screening measures for prostate cancer include the digital rectal examination (DRE) and the prostate-specific antigen (PSA) blood test. Screening may refer to coordinated programs in large populations. *See* Appendix for Cancer Detection Guidelines.

**screening procedure** Any study or examination (blood test, cytology, imaging study, endoscopy) to detect early cancers (and precancerous conditions) before they cause symptoms and are more likely to be cured. Among the most successful screening procedures are the Pap test, mammography, colonoscopy, and prostate-specific antigen (PSA) blood test. *See* Appendix for Cancer Detection Guidelines.

**second-look surgery** A repeat surgical procedure used to carefully examine the abdomen (laparotomy) and to identify and possibly remove persistent or recurrent cancer. It is advised in some cases of colorectal and ovarian cancers. An increase in the blood level of the tumor markers CEA following colon cancer surgery and of CA 125 after ovarian cancer surgery indicate recurrent tumor that often can be successfully treated. Laparoscopy that examines the abdomen using a laparoscope through the abdominal skin and muscles in some cases may be advised instead of laparotomy.

**secondary cancer** A cancer that results from prior therapy, usually chemotherapy or radiation therapy given for a previous unrelated malignancy. As more people with malignant disease, especially children, are living longer following successful treatment, the possibility of secondary cancer has greatly increased. Anyone successfully treated for cancer needs to be followed regularly to detect and treat either a secondary cancer, or a second primary cancer not attributable to prior treatment. *See also* Secondary Primary Cancer.

**second primary cancer** A new cancer occurring in someone with a previous malignancy, which is not attributed to prior chemotherapy, radiation, or other therapy. It is important to distinguish a second primary cancer from a recurrence of the first cancer, because treatment will often be different. The second primary cancer may be of the same type as the first (a new cancer in the opposite breast or in a different area of the colon) or in a different organ. *See also* Secondary Cancer.

**segmental resection** *See* Segmentectomy.

**segmentectomy** Surgical removal of part (segment) of a lobe in an organ; used most often for treating lung and liver cancer. Pulmonary (lung) segmentectomy is usually reserved for people with lung cancer who cannot tolerate the loss of additional lung tissue, as in pulmonary lobectomy. Also called segmental resection. *See also* Liver Cancer (pages 178–179); Lung Cancer (pages 180–182).

**seizure** A sudden episode with loss of consciousness and uncontrolled movements, including loss of bladder and bowel control; often the first indication of a brain tumor. *See also* Brain Tumor (pages 157–159).

**self-examination** A hands-on physical examination of one's body; extremely useful in detecting early breast cancer in women and skin cancer in women and men. Monthly self-examinations should be practiced to detect small malignancies before they cause symptoms and are more likely to be successfully treated. *See* Appendix for Cancer Detection Guidelines; Breast Self-Examination.

**seminoma** A malignant germ cell tumor of young men, which usually occurs in the testes and less often in the mediastinum (chest). It is very responsive to radiation therapy. *See also* Testicular Cancer (pages 206–207).

℞ **Semustine®** *See* Nitrosourea and Methyl-CCNU.

℞ **Senexon®** *See* Senna.

℞ **senna** Also known by the trade names Senexon® and Senokot®, this is a laxative used for the treatment of constipation.

℞ **Senokot®** *See* Senna.

**sentinel node** Lymph node(s) closest to a malignant tumor and considered to be the first site of metastasis (spread); identified using blue dye and/or radioisotope-tagged material injected into skin surrounding the tumor. The injected substance spreads through lymphatics to the adjacent (regional) node area(s) and identifies the sentinel node by color or radioactivity (using a gamma ray-detector). The identified node is removed and examined for cancer cells. If malignant cells are present, then all remaining adjacent (regional) nodes are removed by lymphadenectomy; otherwise the nodes are left in place. The procedure is now used for melanoma, except for very thin and very thick lesions, and is increasingly being used in breast cancer. *See also* Breast Cancer (pages 159–161); Melanoma (pages 182–184).

**sequential excision** *See* Limited Breast Surgery.

℞ **Serax®** *See* Oxazepam.

**serotonin** A natural hormone produced by different tissues, especially platelets, which affects smooth muscle and causes constriction or narrowing of blood vessels and stimulates peristalsis (movement) of stomach and intestines. Excess serotonin produced by carcinoid tumor is responsible for the carcinoid syndrome.

℞ **sertraline hydrochloride** Also known by the trade name Zoloft®, this belongs to a group of drugs known as antidepressants.

**serum** The clear, pale-yellow fluid that separates from coagulated (clotted) blood.

℞ **Serzone®** *See* Nefazodone Hydrochloride.

**shunt** An artificial connection to divert fluid. The Denver® and LeVeen shunts are devices used to remove malignant ascites (abdominal fluid caused by cancer), which causes abdominal swelling and discomfort and interferes with breathing. Shunts are also used to drain fluid from the brain into other locations in the body. *See also* Ascites; Denver® Shunt; LeVeen Shunt; Paracentesis.

**side effect** Any treatment result other than the desired goal of the treatment; most often used to mean an adverse, unwanted, or undesirable effect, which may vary from insignificant to life-threatening. Cancer treatment, particularly with chemotherapy, often causes side effects, the most noticeable being nausea and alopecia (loss of hair); and the most serious being injury to bone marrow, heart, or lungs. In many cases, especially in the very young and old, side effects prevent or at least limit optimal therapy.

**sigmoid colon** The lower part of the colon, shaped like the letter S, which is continuous with the upper portion of the rectum.

**sigmoidoscope** A lighted, tubular, magnifying instrument (endoscope) used to examine and biopsy the interior of the rectum and the sigmoid colon. Also called proctoscope.

**sigmoidoscopy** Examination of the sigmoid colon using a sigmoidoscope to view and biopsy the interior of the lower colon and rectum. The procedure is invaluable for examining the lower digestive tract for tumor and inflammatory bowel disease. It causes little discomfort, requires only a small enema in preparation, and can be done in a physician's office. Also called flexible sigmoidoscopy. *See* Appendix for Cancer Detection Guidelines.

**simulation** A process involving special x-ray pictures that are used to plan radiation treatment so that the area to be treated is precisely located and marked for treatment.

**Sinequan®** *See* Doxepin Hydrochloride.

**Sipple's syndrome** *See* Multiple Endocrine Neoplasia.

**small bowel** The small bowel or small intestine is part of the digestive tract that begins at the pylorus (stomach outlet) and ends at the cecum, which is the first part of the large intestine or colon, where food is mixed with bile and other enzymes and broken down into simple compounds to be absorbed. *See* Small Intestine Cancer (pages 201–202).

**small cell carcinoma** A rapidly growing malignant tumor, when viewed under the microscope, it appears to be made up of cells of uniform small size. Although this rapidly spreading cancer most often arises in the lungs, it can affect the esophagus, prostate, and vagina. About 20% of all primary lung malignancies are small cell (SCLC), which occurs more often in women than men. Unfortunately, SCLC is seldom curable. *See also* Lung Cancer (pages 180–182).

**snuff** Finely-powdered, cured tobacco placed between the gum and cheek (dipped); associated with cancer of the mouth and gum. In the past, snuff-related oral cancer was seen most often in older women in the South; but today, due to the promotion of smokeless tobacco, it is seen most often in young males.

**soft tissue sarcoma** *See* Soft Tissue Cancer (pages 202–204).

**solid tumor** Any cancer that begins as a distinct mass or lump in tissue other than lymph tissue, lymph nodes, and bone marrow. These include the following common cancers: lung, colon, breast, prostate, ovary, pancreas, etc.

**sonogram** *See* Sonography.

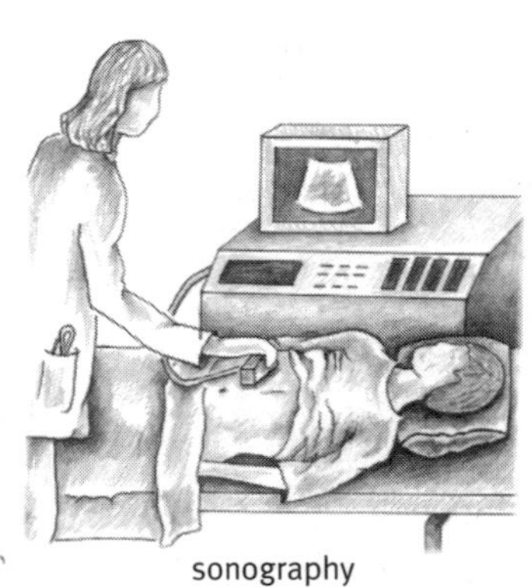

sonography

**sonography** A study using high frequency sound waves to detect, evaluate, and measure structures and tumors deep within the body. A transducer (a small instrument that generates and collects reflected sound waves) is moved over the body, and the collected waves are entered into a computer to produce two-dimensional images or sonograms. The procedure is widely available, safe, and completely painless. Small transducers contained in endoscopes allow examination and staging of tumors of the esophagus and rectum. Sonography is also used to guide needles to biopsy tumors of the breast. Also called ultrasonography.

**sorbitol** This is a sugar known as a hyperosmotic laxative. It is used to treat constipation.

**spinal cord compression** Increased pressure on the spinal cord or nerves in the spine most often caused by cancer that has spread to the bone marrow in a back bone or vertebra, and sometimes by the spread of a tumor to the tissue around the spinal cord. It occurs in up to 5% of people with cancer, and it is second only to brain metastasis as a complication of cancer that has spread to the brain and spinal cord (central nervous system). In a cancer patient, back pain, leg weakness or numbness, or loss of bladder or bowel control indicate a medical emergency requiring prompt treatment. Either immediate surgery to relieve the pressure or irradiation to the spine is needed to prevent permanent paralysis and loss of bladder and bowel control.

**spinal tap** A procedure in which a thin needle is placed in the spinal canal to withdraw a small amount of spinal fluid or to give medicine into the central nervous system through the spinal fluid.

**spleen** The large, lymphatic organ in the left upper part of the abdomen adjacent to the stomach that in early life forms blood and in later life stores both red blood cells and platelets. It filters blood and, as part of the immune system, renders bacteria entering the blood during infection more susceptible to the body's natural defenses. Massive enlargement of the spleen in leukemia, lymphoma, and Hodgkin's disease can cause multiple problems including abdominal pain, hypersplenism (increased removal of platelets from the blood), and splenic rupture, any of which may require splenectomy (removal of the spleen). *See also* Splenectomy.

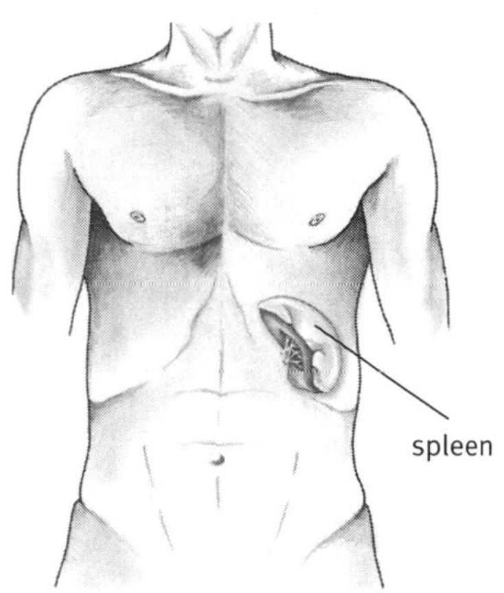


**splenectomy** Surgical removal of the spleen. Whatever the indication, such as cancer or trauma, removal of the spleen, especially in early childhood, causes an individual to become susceptible to certain bacterial infections, especially pneumococcal pneumonia. If possible, individuals undergoing elective splenectomy should receive immunization with pneumococcal vaccine prior to the procedure; if the operation is an emergency or time does not otherwise permit, they should receive the same immunization as soon as practicable following the surgery. Antibiotics should be administered at the first indication of infection (fever, increased numbers of white blood cells) in these patients. *See also* Spleen.

**spontaneous regression** A decrease in size or complete disappearance of a cancer without any treatment (or explanation). It is particularly known to occur in melanoma, kidney cancer, and retinoblastoma.

**sporadic** Any condition or disease, including cancer, which occurs without a family history of repeated, similar disorders, or is not shown to be inherited (passed on or transmitted from parent to offspring).

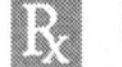
**Sporanox®** *See* Itraconazole.

**spread of cancer** *See* Metastasis.

**squamous cell** A cell when viewed under the microscope that appears flat and similar to a fish scale. Squamous cells are found in many normal tissues, including skin, and lining of the larynx, esophagus, anus, and cervix. *See also* Epithelium.

**squamous cell carcinoma** A type of cancer that affects body tissues normally lined by squamous epithelium (squamous cells), which includes the skin, larynx, esophagus, anus, and cervix. It also arises in squamous metaplasia (tissue changed to squamous epithelium from other epithelial tissue), which happens in non-small cell lung cancer. Squamous cell cancer is identified by its ability to produce keratin, a protein found in skin, hair, and nails. *See also* Bowen's Disease; Epithelium; Squamous Cell.

**stage of cancer** The extent of cancer, or the process of determining the extent of cancer. With few exceptions, cancers other than carcinoma in situ and other early malignancies need to be staged because treatment depends not only on the type, but also the extent of the neoplasm. Obviously, a very small or limited cancer does not require the same treatment as a larger or more extensive malignancy. Although history taking and careful physical examination suggest the extent of a cancer, a battery of diagnostic studies (the staging workup) is needed to accurately define most malignancies. These studies include blood and other laboratory examinations; imaging studies such as x-rays, CT, and MRI; isotope scans; and endoscopy. An early, small tumor or growth that is unlikely to spread does not need an extensive or complex workup. However, lymphoma and leukemia that affect the entire body, as well as lung cancer and other tumors that spread quickly, need an extensive workup. The exact stage of a solid cancer usually is not determined until surgery when biopsies are obtained of the tumor, lymph nodes, and other tissues. Although there are several different staging methods, the TNM method of the American Joint Committee on Cancer (AJCC) is most often used in the United States. It categorizes 49 different cancers according to the following:

*Tumor:* Derived from the extent (size, depth of growth, grade) of the original (primary) growth. Increasing values—T1, T2, T3, T4—indicate increasing size or depth of invasion of a primary cancer. T0 indicates no original or primary growth identified. Tis is carcinoma in situ.

N*ode:* Obtained from presence or absence and extent of metastasis (spread) to adjacent (regional) lymph nodes. Values—N0, N1, N2, N3,—indicate no spread, and then progressive involvement of lymph nodes.

M*etastasis:* The absence or presence of metastasis (spread) to distant organs or tissues; indicated by M0, M1.

Based upon values assigned to T, N, and M, a cancer is placed in one of five stages:

*Stage 0:* Carcinoma in situ, or very early or minimal tumor that with proper treatment is curable in every case.

*Stages I, II, III:* Cancer between the two extremes as far as extent and potential for cure are concerned.

*Stage IV:* Cancer that is very advanced or widespread, and is usually incurable.

Not only does staging play a vital role in the management of malignant disease, it is necessary in cancer research to ensure that both investigation and comparison of treatment methods are meaningful. Although TNM and other staging methods are continually revised as new diagnostic and imaging methods make staging more precise, some cancer experts believe staging may have become unnecessarily complex, and defining stages (IA, IB) may have little bearing on the outlook or the treatment of malignant disease.

**staging laparotomy** Surgery to examine the abdomen and determine the extent or stage of disease, such as Hodgkin's disease. It includes splenectomy (removal of the spleen), liver biopsy, and selected lymph node biopsy. Today, because of more precise diagnostic studies, staging laporotomy is no longer advised in every case of Hodgkin's disease. *See also* Stage of Cancer; Staging Workup.

**staging workup** The process of obtaining diagnostic studies necessary to stage or determine the extent of cancer. Needed studies include blood and laboratory examinations, x-ray and imaging studies (CT, MRI, isotope scan), endoscopy, and biopsies. *See also* Stage of Cancer.

**stem cell** A primitive cell able to reproduce itself and capable of developing into different cell types. Hematopoietic stem cells in the bone marrow give rise to red blood cells, platelets, and granulocytes, a type of white blood cells. Embryonic stem cells give rise to any cell type in the body.

**stem cell transplant** A hematopoietic stem cell graft in which the source of the cells is the patient's (and sometimes another individual's) blood or bone marrow. Umbilical cord blood is also a source. *See also* Bone Marrow Transplant.

**stenosis** A stricture (narrowing) of a duct, canal, or blood vessel.

**stent** A slender metal or plastic tube placed in a tubular structure to overcome obstruction. Stenting of the common bile duct is used to relieve obstruction of bile flow from the liver due to pancreatic cancer; and stenting of the ureter is used to overcome obstruction of urine from the kidney due to cancer in the pelvic area.



**stereotactic breast biopsy** A technique for biopsying breast lumps that cannot be felt, which uses a large needle directed under imaging (x-ray or ultrasound) to obtain a core of tissue. It is useful in some cases in which calcifications or a mass can be seen on a mammogram, but cannot be found by touch. The procedure, which is done under local anesthesia and does not require a surgical incision, is in many instances replacing open or excisional biopsy that removes a part of or the entire mass. *See also* Biopsy.

**stereotactic radiosurgery** A new treatment that focuses high doses of radiation at a tumor while limiting the exposure that normal tissue receives. The treatment may be useful for tumors that are in places where regular surgery would harm essential tissue (in the brain or spinal cord) or where the patient's condition does not permit regular surgery. Also called Gamma knife.

**steroids** A large variety of substances that includes many hormones and drugs having a particular chemical structure in common. It is most often used as a generic term to describe drugs similar to cortisone. Also, a term used by athletes to describe anabolic steroids (that enhance performance by increasing muscle size), which have been banned because of their association with both noncancerous and malignant liver tumors. *See also* Cortisone.

**Stewart-Treves syndrome** A type of angiosarcoma (soft tissue cancer) affecting lymphatics and small blood vessels in the skin of severely swollen arms (lymphedema) in women who have had a mastectomy and often radiation therapy to the lymph nodes under the arm (axilla). *See also* Lymphedema; Mastectomy; Sarcoma; Soft Tissue Cancer (pages 202–204).

℞ **STI-571** Also known by the trade names Gleevec® and Glivec®, this drug is used for the treatment of chronic myelogenous leukemia. It has also been shown to be effective against a rare stomach cancer called "gastrointestinal stromal tumors" and in some cases of acute lymphocytic leukemia. This drug is a signal transduction inhibitor that interferes with defective enzymes, such as bcr/abl and c-kit, which result in the uncontrolled growth (abnormal cell division) of tumor cells.

**stoma** An artificial passage or opening between the skin and a hollow organ, which may be either temporary or permanent. It is designated by the suffix -ostomy, such as colostomy (colon), cystostomy (bladder), ileostomy (ileum), or gastrostomy (stomach). *See* Ostomy.

**stomach** *See* Stomach Cancer (pages 204–206).

**stomal therapist** A health professional trained to care for patients with a stoma (artificial opening) between the skin and intestinal or urinary tract, who provides instruction in diet, skin care, and management of bags (appliances) to collect urine and solid waste. *See also* Stoma.

**stomatitis** Inflammation of the lining of the mouth that often leads to painful oral ulcers and even severe infection. It is often caused by chemotherapy and radiation therapy to the head and neck. All people who receive head and neck radiation, and almost half of those who receive chemotherapy, develop significant oral irritation so painful as to limit their food intake. Treatment includes saline and antacid mouthwash, oral anesthetic solutions, and antibiotics in case of infection.

℞ **streptomycin** This is an antibiotic that belongs to a group of drugs known as aminoglycosides.

℞ **streptozocin** Also known by the trade name Zanosar®, this drug is a nitrosourea belonging to a group of drugs known as alkylating agents. It is used in the treatment of several types of cancer, including carcinoid tumors and pancreatic cancer.

**strontium-89** A radioactive substance that is used for the treatment of bone pain due to metastatic prostate cancer. It is injected into a vein and is attracted to areas of bone containing metastatic cancer. The radiation given off by this substance kills the cancer cells and relieves the pain caused by the bone metastases. *See also* Prostate Cancer (pages 194–196); Radiation Therapy.

**subcutaneous** Relating to the fatty tissue layer beneath the skin. A subcutaneous injection is medication injected by needle into the subcutaneous tissue.

℞ **Sumycin®** *See* Tetracycline Hydrochloride.

**superficial** Situated near the surface of the skin or the lining of an organ. Superficial cancer is a very early-stage malignancy likely to be cured with minimal treatment.

**superficial spreading melanoma** *See* Melanoma (pages 182–184).

**superior pulmonary sulcus tumor** *See* Pancoast Tumor.

**superior vena cava** *See* Vena Cava.

**superior vena cava syndrome (SVCS)** Symptoms due to blockage of the large vein (superior vena cava) in the chest leading to the heart. This syndrome can cause shortness of breath, a full feeling in the head, and a bluish discoloration and swelling of the face and arms. Obstruction of blood from the upper body is most often caused by advanced cancer in the chest, including lung cancer and lymphoma, as well as by cancer spread to the chest, such as breast cancer. Because SVCS is a very serious problem, the exact cause must be determined quickly so that proper therapy with multidrug chemotherapy and/or radiation therapy is not delayed. Bed rest with the head raised, oxygen, cortisone-like medication, and diuretics are used as immediate therapy.

**suppression of bone marrow** *See* Myelosuppression.

**Suprax®** *See* Cefixime.

**surgical therapy** Surgery remains the cornerstone for controlling most solid cancers (tumors due to malignant disease other than leukemia, myeloma, lymphoma, and Hodgkin's disease). Except in the cases of very early-stage tumors, the usual cancer operation removes the original or primary growth together with surrounding normal tissue and adjacent (regional) lymph nodes. Today, for malignancies such as breast, and head and neck cancers, surgery combined with radiation therapy and chemotherapy enables smaller operations to give results equal to those previously obtained by larger and more extensive procedures. In some instances, cancer that has metastasized to the lung or liver, which was once considered incurable, can be removed and permanently controlled.

Not only is surgery the primary means of curing most solid cancers, it is also invaluable in diagnosing and determining the stage (extent) of malignant disease, providing vein access for giving chemotherapy and other medications, relieving intestinal and urinary obstruction, relieving or lessening pain and other symptoms, and rehabilitating patients following cancer treatment.

**survival rate** The percentage of people who live a certain period of time. The 5-year survival rate refers to the percentage of patients who live at least 5 years after diagnosis, and the 5-year rates are used to produce a standard way of discussing prognosis. Five-year survival rates exclude from calculations patients dying of other diseases; considered to be a more accurate way to describe the prognosis for patients with a particular type and stage of cancer. *See also* Five-Year Survival Rate.

**symptom** Any complaint or difficulty that is a sign or indication of an underlying medical problem or disease.

**synchronous** At the same time (cancer in both breasts at the same time).

**syndrome** A group of varied symptoms that together characterize or indicate a particular medical condition, such as acquired immunodeficiency syndrome (AIDS).

**Synercid®** *See* Quinupristin and Dalfopristin.

**synovial sarcoma** A rare type of cancer involving the synovium (soft tissue lining the joint), which usually occurs around the knee in young adults. Unlike other soft tissue sarcomas, these tumors can be painful. *See also* Sarcoma; Soft Tissue Cancer (pages 202–204).

# T

℞ **Tabloid®** *See* Thioguanine.

℞ **tamoxifen** Also known by the trade name Nolvadex®, this oral antiestrogen drug is used to treat women with breast cancer that is estrogen receptor positive (tumor growth is influenced by the female hormone estrogen). Depending on the size of the cancer and whether it has spread to lypmh nodes, tamoxifen may be used alone or together with chemotherapy.

Tamoxifen has also been approved for women of all ages at high risk for developing breast cancer (previous cancer in the opposite breast, a strong family history, presence of mutant BRCA genes) to reduce their chance of developing cancer.

Although the drug blocks estrogen's effect on breast tissue, in other situations it mimics estrogen by strengthening bones and lowering blood cholesterol. About 25% of women taking tamoxifen experience hot flashes, mild nausea, and vomiting; however, very few experience more serious side effects, such as blood clots. Because it slightly increases the risk of endometrial cancer, women who take the drug should be monitored carefully for any evidence of uterine cancer, such as vaginal bleeding and vaginal discharge. After starting the medication, some women with breast cancer involving bone may notice a temporary flare (increase in bone pain), which usually indicates the malignancy is responding to treatment. *See also* Breast Cancer (pages 159–161).

℞ **Targretin®** *See* Bexarotene.

℞ **Taxol®** *See* Paclitaxel.

℞ **Taxotere®** *See* Docetaxel.

℞ **Tazicef®** *See* Ceftazidime.

℞ **Tazidime®** *See* Ceftazidime.

℞ **Tazocin®** *See* Piperacillin Sodium Combined with Tazobactam Sodium.

**T cell** A variety of lymphocyte or white blood cell that is part of the body's immune (protective) system. All subtypes of T cells, including suppressor cells and helper cells, develop in the thymus gland in the chest from stem cells that originate in the bone marrow and migrate in the blood to the thymus. Cellular immunity (the ability of T cells to protect the body by engulfing infected cells) is being investigated as cancer therapy. T cell malignancies include some forms of leukemia and lymphoma in both children and adults.

**technetium-99m** A manufactured radioisotope used to make scans (images) of internal organs, including bone, brain, liver, thyroid, lung, kidney, heart. More recently, it has been used to identify the sentinel node(s) in melanoma and breast cancer. Technetium-99m has a half-life of 6 hours (it loses half its radioactivity in 6 hours, after which the remaining half of the original radioactivity decays in 6 hours, and so on).

℞ **Tegafur®** *See* UFT (Ftorafur and Uracil).

**teletherapy** *See* External Beam Radiation.

℞ **teniposide** Also known as VM-26 and by the trade name Vumon®, this drug belongs to a group of drugs known as plant alkaloids. It is an inhibitor of topoisomerase, and is used in the treatment of several types of cancer, including leukemias and lymphomas.

**TEP** *See* Tracheoesophageal Puncture.

**teratoma** A tumor containing several types of tissue not normally part of the organ in which the growth arises. Teratomas occur in many parts of the body, most frequently in the ovary, where they are usually not malignant, and less commonly in the testis, where they are often cancerous.

**testicle** The primary male sex glands, located in the scrotum or sac beneath the penis. *See* Testicular Cancer (pages 206–207).

**testicular** Relating to the testicle or testis. *See* Testicular Cancer (pages 206–207).

**testis** *See* Testicle.

**testosterone** The most potent male hormone, which is produced mainly in the testicles or testes and possibly in the adrenal gland (adrenal cortex) and other sites.

℞ **tetracycline hydrochloride** Also known by the trade names Achromycin®, Panmycin®, and Sumycin®, this drug is an antibiotic that belongs to the group of drugs known as tetracyclines.

℞ **thalidomide** Also known by the trade name Thalomid®, this drug used to be prescribed as a sedative; however, it caused severe birth defects and was withdrawn from the market. Currently, it is used to increase appetite, weight, and body mass in patients with cancer-related cachexia (loss of appetite, weight, and body mass). It is also useful in the treatment of patients with multiple myeloma.

℞ **Thalomid®** *See* Thalidomide.

**therapy** Any treatment of disease or medical disorder.

℞ **thiethylperazine** Also known by the trade name Torecan®, this drug belongs to a group of drugs known as phenothiazines. It is used to treat nausea and vomiting caused by chemotherapy.

℞ **thioguanine** Also known by the trade name Tabloid®, this drug belongs to a group of drugs known as antimetabolites. It is used to treat several types of cancer, including leukemia.

℞ **Thioplex®** *See* Thiotepa.

℞ **thiotepa** Also known by the trade name Thioplex®, this alkylating-type of chemotherapy drug has been used to treat cancer for almost 50 years. Given intravenously in high doses, it is used with bone marrow transplant to treat leukemia, Hodgkin's disease, and breast cancer. Instilled into the bladder, it is useful in treating early-stage bladder cancer. The main adverse effect is granulocytopenia (bone marrow toxicity that lowers the number of white blood cells in blood).

**thoracentesis** Needle puncture of the chest to remove fluid (pleural effusion) between the lung and inside of the chest. Malignant pleural effusion from lung cancer and malignancies that have spread to the lung (breast cancer) often builds up rapidly and requires immediate drainage to relieve shortness of breath. Thoracentesis is also used to diagnose and stage lung cancer by identifying cancer cells in pleural fluid.

**thoracoscope** A lighted, magnifying instrument (endoscope) used to examine the inside of the chest (and lung). It is introduced between the ribs.

**thoracoscopy** Endoscopy using a thoracoscope inserted in the chest under general anesthesia. It is used to view the interior of the chest, biopsy lung and pleura (chest lining), and strip pleura from the inside of the chest.

**thoracotomy** A major surgical procedure performed under general anesthesia to open the thorax (chest) to gain access to the lungs and other chest organs. Exploratory thoracotomy is used to diagnose and evaluate chest and lung cancers for possible removal, and in many instances has been replaced by thoracoscopy, a much less invasive procedure. *See also* Lung Cancer (pages 180–182).

**thorax** The upper part of the body between the neck and abdomen that contains the organs of respiration (trachea, lungs) and circulation (heart, pulmonary arteries, veins).

℞ **Thorazine®** *See* Chlorpromazine.

**three-dimensional conformal therapy** This treatment uses sophisticated computers to precisely map the location of the cancer within the prostate. The patient is filled with a plastic mold, resembling a body cast, to keep him still so the radiation can be more accurately aimed. Radiation beams are then aimed from several directions. *See also* Prostate Cancer (pages 194–196); Radiation Therapy.

**thrombocyte** *See* Platelet.

**thrombocytopenia** Decreased numbers of thrombocytes (platelets) in blood that, when severe, can result in excessive bleeding, especially following surgery. Malignancy involving the spleen (lymphoma, Hodgkin's disease, leukemia) can cause hypersplenism that results in thrombocytopenia. Also, many chemotherapy drugs suppress production of platelets in the bone marrow, which results in varying degrees of thrombocytopenia. Immediate treatment is platelet transfusion.

**thrombocytosis** Increased numbers of thrombocytes (platelets) in the blood that can lead to blood clots. It is a common manifestation (paraneoplastic syndrome) of cancer, especially Hodgkin's disease, lymphoma, and leukemia. It is also an adverse effect of leucovorin.

**thrombophlebitis** Inflammation of a vein that often causes blood clots that result in swelling of an arm or leg. It may be the first symptom of an unsuspected cancer, especially of the pancreas, particularly if it is migratory (involves more than one vein). Deep venous thrombophlebitis (DVT) of pelvic veins can dislodge blood clots to the lungs that may be fatal. Treatment of thrombophlebitis includes elevating the limb on pillows, bed rest, and anticoagulants (heparin, warfarin) that delay blood clotting. Thrombophlebitis associated with cancer usually persists or returns unless the malignancy is controlled. *See also* Heparin; Warfarin.

**thrush** A fungal infection of the mouth due to Candida albicans often causes stomatitis (painful mouth ulcers). It can result from cancer chemotherapy, and conditions such as AIDS that depress the body's immune (protective) mechanism. Treatment is with an antifungal antibiotic medication (nystatin) rinsed in the mouth.

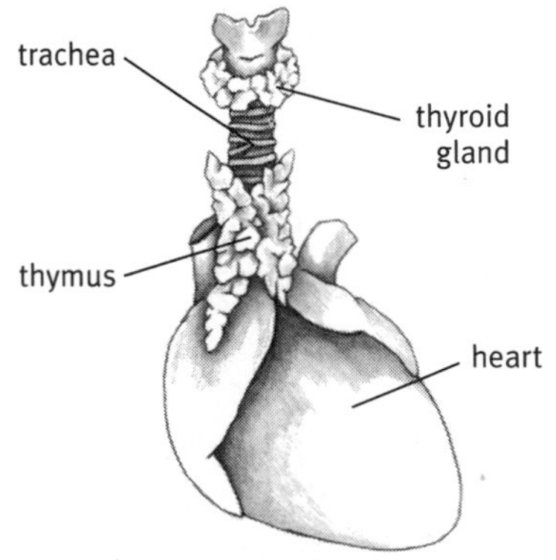


**thymus** A gland-like organ in the upper part of the chest beneath the sternum (breast bone) made up of lymphatic tissue. It produces T cells (thymus-derived cells), a type of white blood cell or lymphocyte vital to the body's immune (protective) mechanism. The gland may be a site of thymoma, a generally benign (noncancerous) tumor associated with myasthenia gravis (a disease of progressive muscular weakness), as well as thymic carcinoma, a generally fast growing cancer with a poor outlook.

**thyrocalcitonin** *See* Calcitonin.

**thyroid** The thyroid is a hormone-producing (endocrine) gland in the front of the neck that produces several hormones that regulate metabolism (chemical and physical processes that control the body's growth and energy). *See* Thyroid Cancer (pages 207–209).

**thyroid-stimulating hormone** A hormone produced by the pituitary gland in the base (under surface) of the brain, which controls the growth and function of the thyroid gland. Also called TSH.

℞ **Ticar®** *See* Ticarcillin Disodium.

℞ **ticarcillin disodium** Also known by the trade name Ticar®, this drug is an antibiotic that belongs to a general group of drugs known as semi-synthetic penicillins.

**tissue** Groups of similar cells and substances surrounding them that together make up an organ. The four basic body tissues are epithelial tissue—skin, lining of organs, and glands; connective tissue—bone, cartilage, and blood; nerve; and muscle.

**TNM staging** A method for determining the stage or extent of cancer based on the involvement of a tumor at the primary site (T), adjacent (regional) lymph node spread (N), and distant spread (M). It is one of many staging systems to determine the required treatment and predict outcome. *See* Stage of Cancer.

℞ **tobramycin sulfate** Also known by the trade name Nebcin®, this is an antibiotic that belongs to a group of drugs known as aminoglycosides.

℞ **Tofranil-PM®** *See* Imipramine Pamoate.

℞ **topotecan** Also known by the trade name Hycamtin®, this intravenous chemotherapy drug is used to treat recurrent ovarian cancer and small cell lung cancer. Its main unwanted side effect is bone marrow toxicity with decreased numbers of white blood cells and platelets in the blood. It also causes fever and flu-like symptoms.

℞ **Toradol®** *See* Ketorolac Tromethamine.

℞ **Torecan®** *See* Thiethylperazine.

℞ **toremifene** Also known by the trade name Fareston®, this oral drug, similar to tamoxifen (Nolvadex®), is used to treat advanced-stage breast cancer in postmenopausal women with either estrogen-receptor positive or unknown-receptor tumors.

 **tositumomab** Also known by the trade name Bexxar®, this is a radioimmunotherapeutic agent composed of a monoclonal antibody with a radioactive substance (iodine-131) attached to it. It is directed to a specific receptor (CD20) located on B lymphocytes and is used in the treatment of non-Hodgkin's lymphoma.

**total parenteral nutrition (TPN)** A technique used to either supplement or provide complete nutrition by means of intravenous (IV) fluids. Solutions containing protein in the form of amino acids, fats, carbohydrates, vitamins, and minerals furnish all nutrients necessary for the body's energy, growth, and repair. TPN can be life saving for patients unable to eat due to cancer or cancer treatment. Because most solutions contain large amounts of carbohydrates that cause phlebitis (inflamed veins), TPN must be given through a vascular access device. Although long-term parenteral nutrition sometimes is given outside the hospital, it remains an expensive, complex procedure requiring constant care and monitoring. Common problems include bacterial infection and chemical imbalance, especially sugar, sodium, potassium, chloride, calcium, and magnesium.

**TPN** *See* Total Parenteral Nutrition.

**trachea** The large air tube or windpipe in the neck and upper chest that extends from the throat to the carina where it divides into a left and right mainstem bronchus to each lung.

**tracheoesophageal puncture** A surgical procedure used to restore the voice after laryngectomy (removal of the larynx). A small device placed in the trachea (windpipe) in the neck enables postlaryngectomy patients to speak without placing a buzzing instrument against the neck.

**tracheotomy** An operation to create a stoma (opening) in the trachea (windpipe) in the neck. A temporary tracheotomy is used to relieve blockage of airflow in head and neck trauma, and to provide an airway when a respirator is required for long periods. Permanent tracheotomy is necessary following laryngectomy (total removal of the larynx).

 **Transderm-SCOP®** *See* Scopolamine.

**transillumination** *See* Diaphanography.

**transitional cell** A type of cell lining the urinary collecting system (kidney, ureter, bladder). Also called urothelial cell.

**transvaginal ultrasonography** An imaging study using ultrasound generated by a tube-like device in the vagina, which permits the detection of most ovarian cancers.

**transverse colon** The second section of the colon. It is called the transverse colon because it crosses the body from the upper right part of the abdomen to the left part of the abdomen. *See also* Colon.

℞ **trastuzumab** Also known by the trade name Herceptin®, this anticancer drug is a monoclonal antibody specific for the HER2/*neu* gene. It is used alone or in combination with other chemotherapy to treat metastatic (widespread) breast cancer that tests positive for abnormal activity (overexpression) of the HER2/*neu* gene detected by laboratory tests. The most severe unwanted side effect is cardiomyopathy (injury to the heart).

℞ **trazodone hydrochloride** Also known by the trade name Desyrel®, this drug belongs to the group of drugs known as antidepressants.

℞ **tretinoin** Also known by the trade name Vesanoid®, this is a derivative of vitamin A. It is used to treat acute promyelocytic leukemia.

℞ **Trilafon®** *See* Perphenazine.

℞ **Trilisate®** *See* Choline Magnesium Trisalicylate.

℞ **trimetrexate** Also known by the trade name Neutrexin®, this drug belongs to a group of drugs known as antimetabolites. It is used in the treatment of several types of cancer, including colon cancer. It is also used to treat a bacterial infection (*Pneumocystis carinii* pneumonia) in individuals with low immune function.

℞ **trovafloxacin** Also known by the trade name Trovan®, this drug is an antibiotic that belongs to a group of drugs known as fluoroquinolones.

℞ **Trovan®** *See* Trovafloxacin.

**Trucut needle** A large bore, hollow biopsy needle that provides a core of material much larger than a tissue sample obtained with fine needle aspiration. It is used to biopsy prostate, liver, and large tumors in breast and limbs. *See also* Biopsy.

**trunk** Part of the body other than head and extremities (arms and legs), which consists of the chest and abdomen. Also called torso.

**TSH** *See* Thyroid-Stimulating Hormone.

**tube** *See* Fallopian Tube.

**tubular carcinoma** A special type of low-grade infiltrating breast cancer that accounts for approximately 2% of invasive breast cancers. The prognosis for this type of cancer is considered to be better than average. *See also* Breast Cancer (pages 159–161).

**tumor** Literally a swollen area; most often used to indicate a new growth, particularly a solid cancer that is causing a lump or mass. *See* Neoplasm; Malignancy.

**tumor board** A group of physicians and health care professionals in a hospital or cancer center who meet regularly to discuss and make treatment recommendations regarding cancer patients presented to them. The board usually is comprised of medical, radiation, and surgical oncologists, radiologists, pathologists, and nurses.

**tumor dose** The cumulative amount of radiation delivered in fractional (divided) doses to cancer during radiation therapy; measured in either grays (Gys) or rads (1 Gy = 100 rads).

**tumor marker** Any one of a number of different, chemical substances in the blood and other body fluids used to detect and identify different cancers. These substances, produced either by a cancer or the body's response to a malignancy, are also used to indicate tumor burden (size of tumor) before treatment, monitor response to therapy, and identify early recurrence. The ideal tumor marker should be 100% specific (occurs only with a particular cancer) and 100% sensitive (present in every case of the cancer). Although markers are neither totally specific nor sensitive, they are useful in gauging the effect of therapy and in indicating recurrent cancer before symptoms occur. Prostate-specific antigen (PSA) is used widely as a screening procedure to detect early prostate cancer before it causes symptoms, when it is more likely to be controlled.

Among the most common tumor markers are PSA—prostate; CEA (carcinoembryonic antigen)—colon, rectum; CA 125 (cancer antigen 125)—ovary; CA 19-9 (cancer antigen 19-9)—pancreas; AFP (alpha-fetoprotein)—liver, testicle; hCG (human chorionic gonadotropin)—ovary, testicle, mediastinum.

It is important to realize the shortcomings of many common markers used to detect cancer or to predict a likelihood of difficulty at a later date. PSA may be elevated very slightly following a simple finger rectal examination or up to 48 hours following sexual activity. CEA (which is usually used to follow a patient with cancer, rather than as a screening test) is often increased in cigarette smokers. BRCA indicates a likelihood of breast cancer and ovarian cancer in only a small number (5%) of women. In light of this, anyone having a having a blood test for a marker to detect or predict the likelihood of cancer should have the possible results and implications of the test carefully explained before the test is done.

**tumor necrosis factor** A naturally occurring hormone produced in minute amounts by macrophages (large cells produced in bone marrow) that surround and destroy bacteria in tissue. Because tumor necrosis factor can kill tumor cells, it is being evaluated as cancer immunotherapy.

**tumor suppressor genes** Genes that slow down cell division or cause cells to die at the appropriate time. Alterations of these genes can lead to too much cell growth and the development of cancer.

**tylectomy** *See* Limited Breast Surgery.

℞ **Tylenol®** *See* Acetaminophen.

# U

℞ **UFT (ftorafur and uracil)** Also known by the trade name Tegafur®, this drug combination belongs to a group of drugs known as antimetabolites. Ftorafur is metabolized to fluorouracil (5-FU) and uracil is an amino acid that enhances the effect of 5-FU. It is used in the treatment of several types of cancer, including colon cancer.

**ulcerative colitis** A disease of the colon of unknown origin that produces inflammation in the colon and rectum and leads to colonic ulcers, bleeding, infection, and diarrhea. Extensive chronic (long standing) ulcerative colitis is linked to a greatly increased risk of colorectal cancer. Patients must be followed carefully, even if they have no clinical evidence of active disease. *See also* Crohn's Disease; Inflammatory Bowel Disease.

**ultrasonography** *See* Sonography.

**umbilical cord** The structure containing blood vessels that connect an unborn infant to the placenta (afterbirth) attached to the inside of the uterus of the mother. Blood from the placenta is used as a source of stem cells in stem cell transplant. *See* Bone Marrow Transplant.

℞ **Unasyn®** *See* Ampicillin Sodium Combined with Sulbactam.

**undifferentiated cancer** *See* Anaplastic Cancer.

**unilateral** Affecting one side of the body. For example, unilateral breast cancer occurs in one breast only.

℞ **Unipen®** *See* Nafcillin Sodium.

**unproven treatment** This is a treatment that has little basis in scientific fact in that there is inadequate scientific evidence available to support its use. Relying on this type of treatment alone, and avoiding conventional medical care, may have serious health consequences. *See also* Alternative Therapy.

**urethral stricture** A narrowing of the urethra due to scar tissue that blocks the flow of urine and can result in overflow incontinence. This can be treated by surgically removing the scar tissue or by stretching (dilating) the urethra.

**urine cytology** Examination of urine under a microscope to look for cancerous and precancerous cells.

**urothelial cell** *See* transitional cell.

**uterine** Pertaining to the uterus (womb).

**uterine cancer** *See* Endometrial Cancer (pages 165–167).

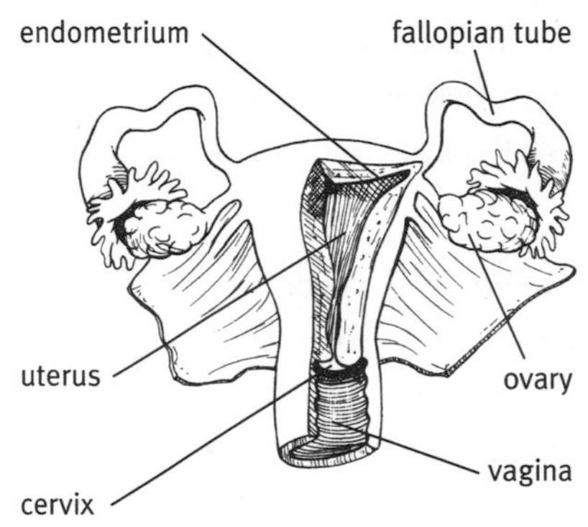


**uterus** The small, hollow, female organ of reproduction in the pelvic area, about the size and shape of a pear. It is lined with tissue (endometrium) to which a fertilized egg from the ovary attaches and develops into an embryo. The lower end or cervix (neck) is where the uterus joins the upper portion of the birth canal or vagina. Also called womb. *See* Endometrial Cancer (pages 165–167).

**uterus cancer** *See* Endometrial Cancer (pages 165–167).

**uveal melanoma** This rare eye cancer develops in the uvea, or middle tissue (iris, ciliary body, and choroid) of the eye, that contains blood vessels and includes the iris that gives the eye its color. Although it accounts for only about 3% of all melanomas, it is the most common malignant tumor of the eye. Unlike cutaneous melanoma (melanoma of the skin), it is not becoming more common. People who develop uveal melanoma are most likely to be in their 60s and white. Caucasians are eight times more likely than African Americans to develop the tumor. The cancer spreads first inside the eyeball or globe, then to tissues surrounding the eye, and later through blood to distant sites, particularly the liver.

Symptoms range from vision problems in early-stage disease, to eye pain in advanced cases. The diagnosis is made by examining the interior of the eye through the pupil by means of a lighted, magnifying instrument (ophthalmoscope), and the extent of disease is often determined with sonography. In the past, the usual treatment for uveal melanoma was removal of the eye or enucleation; but today, removal of the tumor combined with radiation therapy enables some sight to be preserved in certain cases. Also called ocular melanoma.

# V

**vaccine** A fluid preparation made from live, weakened, or killed microscopic organisms, either whole or fragmented. It is used to immunize (protect) against infectious diseases. Among the diseases prevented by immunization are those caused by bacteria—whooping cough, diphtheria, tetanus, and pneumonia; and viruses—smallpox, influenza, measles, hepatitis A and B, and rabies.

Tumor vaccines made from malignant cells grown in tissue culture, which stimulate the body's immune system, have been developed against some cancers, but none have been approved for general use in the United States. Although favorable responses have been reported with melanoma vaccines, the excellent results obtained with infectious disease vaccines have not been realized with vaccines directed against cancer. At this time, these anticancer agents remain under investigation. However, in the future, preparations made from genetically altered cancer cells grown in the laboratory may generate stronger immune responses and provide greater control over malignancies.

**vagina** The birth canal; part of the female reproductive system that connects the lower portion of the uterus (womb) to the vulva (external female genitals). *See* Vaginal Cancer (pages 209–211).

**vaginal** Pertaining to the vagina or birth canal.

℞ **valacyclovir hydrochloride** Also known by the trade name Valtrex®, this drug belongs to a group of drugs known as antiviral agents. It is used to treat infections with herpesvirus, herpes zoster virus, Epstein-Barr virus, and cytamegalovirus.

℞ **Valium®** *See* Diazepam.

℞ **valspodar** Also known by the trade name Amdray®, this drug is a chemotherapy sensitizer. Some cancer cells have a gene that allows the cells to get rid of chemotherapeutic drugs; thus, the cells are not damaged by the chemotherapy. A chemotherapy sensitizer prevents the cell from eliminating the chemotherapy. Valspodar binds to the surface of the cancer cell and prevents the gene from removing the chemotherapeutic drug when it enters the cell.

℞ **Valtrex®** *See* Valacyclovir Hydrochloride.

℞ **Vancocin®** *See* Vancomycin Hydrochloride.

℞ **vancomycin hydrochloride** Also known by the trade name Vancocin®, this drug is an antibiotic. It is useful in treating a number of different types of bacterial infections, especially those caused by staphylococci.

**vascular access device** A small plastic tube secured in a vein, which enables an individual to receive prolonged or repeated intravenous therapy (total parenteral nutrition [TPN], chemotherapy) and to have blood sampled without repeated needle sticks of the veins, which are often scarred and difficult to find. Either an external catheter that exits the skin or an implantable port underneath the skin is used. The former is a soft plastic catheter placed in the subclavian vein beneath the collarbone by means of a very minor surgical procedure.

An implantable port consists of a small plastic or metal reservoir (chamber) with a plastic self-sealing window (port) attached to a soft plastic catheter inserted into a subclavian vein. Fluid is given or blood is sampled using a small needle pierced through the skin and port into the chamber. When not in use, the reservoir is filled with heparin to prevent clotting. *See also* Heparin; Implantable Port.

℞ **Vectrin®** *See* Minocycline Hydrochloride.

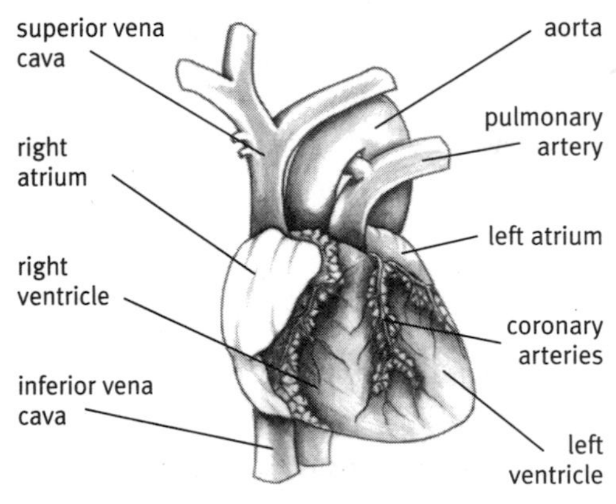


℞ **Velban®** *See* Vinblastine.

℞ **Velosef®** *See* Cephradine.

**vena cava** Either of the two large veins that return blood to the heart. The superior vena cava (SVC) carries blood from the upper body (head, arms, upper part of the chest), and the inferior vena cava (IVC) returns blood from the lower body (lower part of the chest, abdomen, pelvis, legs). Either can (very rarely) be the site of leiomyosarcoma (a type of soft tissue sarcoma). *See also* Superior Vena Cava Syndrome.

℞ **venlafaxine hydrochloride** Also known by the trade name Effexor®, this drug belongs to the group of drugs known as antidepressants.

℞ **Vesanoid®** *See* Tretinoin.

**villous adenoma** A type of adenoma (benign tumor of glandular epithelial tissue) in the lining of the large intestine and sometimes in the duodenum that is a flat, velvety growth. In both locations, it has a high likelihood of becoming cancer—25% in the colon and rectum and 48% in the small intestine. In the large intestine, it often causes rectal bleeding; and in the duodenum, it sometimes blocks flow of bile from the liver and causes jaundice. During endoscopy, the usual villous adenoma is easily recognized as a soft, velvet-like, flat growth. Because of the great tendency of villous adenomas to develop into cancer, all should be surgically removed or completely destroyed by electrocautery (electric current) or laser. Surgical removal is preferred because it enables the entire growth to be examined for cancer, the presence of which requires additional surgery.

℞ **vinblastine** Also known by the trade name Velban®, this chemotherapy drug is used in treating a variety of malignancies including testicular cancer, Hodgkin's disease, Kaposi's sarcoma, lymphomas, and breast cancer. The most serious adverse effect is suppression of bone marrow that results in neutropenia (decreased numbers of white blood cells). It can also cause nerve damage with numbness, tingling, and weakness; but this occurs less frequently than with the related drug vincristine.

**vinca alkaloids** Naturally occurring or semiartificial (semisynthetic) chemical compounds from which cancer chemotherapy drugs (vinblastine, vincristine, vinorelbine) are derived. Vinca alkaloids interfere with microtubules, cellular structures necessary for cell function and growth.

℞ **vincristine** Also known by the trade name Oncovin®, this chemotherapy drug is used in treating many different malignancies including lung, breast, and ovarian cancers, as well as lymphomas, Hodgkin's disease, acute leukemia, and childhood tumors such as Wilms' tumor (nephroblastoma), neuroblastoma, and rhabdomyosarcoma. Its main adverse effect is neurotoxicity (nerve damage) that causes numbness and tingling of the fingers and toes, clumsiness of the hands, constipation, headache, and seizures.

℞ **vindesine** Also known by the trade name Eldisine®, this drug belongs to a group of drugs known as plant alkaloids. It is being studied as a treatment for some types of cancer, including lung cancer.

℞ **vinorelbine** Also known by the trade name Navelbine®, this chemotherapy drug is used for the treatment of non-small cell lung cancer (NSCLC), and it may be useful in breast cancer. It is very corrosive to the surrounding skin and tissue if it extravasates (leaks from a vein), and it can also cause phlebitis (inflamed veins) if administered too slowly.

**vipoma** A tumor, usually found in the pancreas, that produces the hormone-like substance vasoactive intestinal polypeptide, which causes severe watery diarrhea, dehydration, and hypokalemia (low levels of potassium in the blood). The tumor is considered malignant only if it has spread.

**virus** Any one of a great number of very small organisms (usually visible only with an electron microscopy) that reproduce only in a living cell. Viruses are responsible for infectious diseases in humans, including the common cold, flu, measles, hepatitis, polio, and AIDS, as well as in animals and plants. They are also known to cause cancer in cats, birds, rats, and mice. Although viruses have long been suspected to cause malignancy in humans, none have been shown to be the specific cause of human cancer. However, they are known to cause diseases that lead to cancer. Viral hepatitis causing severe liver damage and scarring (cirrhosis) may result in liver cancer. Additionally, viral infection with the human immunodeficiency virus (HIV) that causes AIDS is associated with a number of different malignancies: Kaposi's sarcoma, cervical cancer, and brain lymphoma. *See* Acquired Immunodeficiency Syndrome.

**Vistide®** *See* Cidofovir.

**VM-26** *See* Teniposide.

**vocal cord** Either of two small folds of tissue that are part of the larynx (voice box), whose back and forth movements act like small curtains to produce vocal sounds from air passing in between. In the United States, cancer of the larynx arises in the cords in two-thirds of cases. Motion of each cord is independent and controlled by a recurrent laryngeal nerve. Injury to one nerve, either from trauma during neck operations (especially thyroid surgery) or cancer involving the nerve, results in vocal cord paralysis and hoarseness. Injury to both recurrent laryngeal nerves causes a loss of the voice and difficulty in breathing. *See* Laryngeal Cancer (pages 175–176).

**voice box** *See* Larynx.

**von Recklinghausen disease** *See* Neurofibromatosis.

**VP-16** *See* Etoposide.

**Vumon®** *See* Teniposide.

**vulva** The vulva or external female genitalia comprised of the labia (large and small vaginal lips), clitoris, vaginal opening, and urethra (bladder opening). *See* Vulvar Cancer (pages 211–212).

**vulvar** Relating to the vulva.

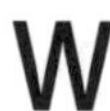

**Waldeyer's ring** Lymphatic tissue in the back of the nose, throat, tonsils, and adenoids.

**warfarin** Also known by the trade name Coumadin®, an anticoagulant drug given by mouth or vein to prevent and treat blood clots in veins. It prolongs coagulation (blood clotting) by interfering with prothrombin, a protein formed and stored in the liver, and the dose of warfarin is adjusted according to the prothrombin time (PT) blood test. Because factors, including medical condition, travel, diet, and medication (alone or combined) influence sensitivity to the drug, people receiving warfarin should have their PT closely monitored, and their physicians should be made aware of all medications (including herbs and other supplements) and medical problems.

**watchful waiting** A term used to describe a physician's decision to closely monitor a disease such as prostate cancer, instead of actively treating the condition. This may be a reasonable choice for older men with small tumors that might grow very slowly. If the situation changes, treatment can be started. *See also* Prostate Cancer (pages 194–196).

℞ **Wellbutrin®** *See* Bupropion Hydrochloride.

**Wermer's syndrome** *See* Multiple Endocrine Neoplasia.

**Whipple operation** The surgical procedure known as pancreaticoduodenectomy, which removes the lower portion of the stomach, gallbladder, lower part of common bile duct, head of pancreas, and duodenum. The operation was developed to treat pancreatic, ampullary, and bile duct cancer. *See also* Ampulla of Vater.

**white blood cell (WBC)** Known medically as a leukocyte, any one of three different cell types: granulocytes from bone marrow; lymphocytes from lymphatic tissue; and monocytes in bone marrow, lymph, and other tissue. They circulate in the blood and act as part of the immune system that protects against microorganisms (bacteria, viruses, fungi). Granulocytes are the most numerous WBCs. They destroy organisms by surrounding and engulfing (digesting) them. Lymphocytes, the second most numerous white blood cells, destroy organisms using antibodies from B lymphocytes and engulf them with T lymphocytes. Monocytes destroy organisms not killed by granulocytes and lymphocytes. Granulocytes are especially sensitive to the toxic effects that many chemotherapy drugs have on bone marrow, which causes granulocytopenia (a reduction in their numbers) and can lead to severe, overwhelming infection.

Leukemia is cancer of leukocyte-forming tissue in which there is uncontrolled growth of abnormal WBCs. It usually produces an increase in their numbers in the blood. There are also leukemias that involve the red blood cell precursors found in the bone marrow, but these are much less common than the leukemias of white blood cells. *See also* Granulocyte; Leukemia (pages 176–178); Lymphocyte.

**Whitmore-Jewett staging system** Classifies prostate cancer as A, B, C, or D. It can be translated into the TNM system. *See also* Stage of Cancer.

**wire localization** A technique used to remove a breast lump that cannot be felt. A wire is guided into a breast mass, by means of mammography or ultrasonography, to identify it for excisional biopsy. In many instances, wire localization has been replaced by stereotactic breast biopsy. *See also* Biopsy.

**womb** *See* Uterus.

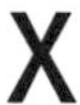

# X

℞ **Xanax®** *See* Alprazolam.

℞ **Xeloda®** *See* Capecitabine.

**xeroderma pigmentosum** A rare, inherited disorder that causes the skin and eyes to be very sensitive to sunlight and leads to skin cancers including melanoma. Total protection from the sun is important for these patients and may decrease the development of skin tumors. Patients with this disorder must be under very careful medical supervision.

**xerostomia** Excessive dryness of the mouth often caused by radiation therapy to the head and neck area, which can accelerate the development of mucositis (painful irritation of mouth, gums, tongue, lips, throat). It also affects taste, which can lead to loss of appetite and sometimes to severe weight loss. Treatment includes good oral hygiene and frequent mouthwash.

**X-linked** Any inherited trait or disorder caused by a gene located on the X (female) chromosome, which includes different syndromes associated with lymphoma, leukemia, and myeloma. *See also* Y-linked.

**x-ray** A type of ionizing radiation produced by an electrical device. It is used to make images of the body and is used in high doses as radiation therapy for cancer. The term is commonly used to mean the picture obtained from x-ray imaging (chest x-ray). Also called Roentgen ray. *See also* Imaging Study.

℞ **Xylocaine®** *See* Lidocaine.

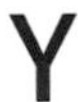

# Y

**YAG laser** A yttrium aluminum garnet laser used to temporarily overcome blockage of the esophagus or bronchus due to advanced cancer that cannot be removed by surgery.

**Y-linked** Any inherited trait or disorder caused by a gene located on the Y chromosome, which is responsible for the male sex. *See also* X-linked.

**yolk sac tumor** The most common malignant germ cell tumor of infants and young children, which occurs most often in the testis or ovary, and less often in the mediastinum (central part of the chest). These tumors arise from remnants of structures present shortly after conception early in the developing embryo. Usual treatment is surgery or radiation therapy and chemotherapy.

# Z

**Zanosar®** *See* Streptozocin.

**Zilactin-B®** A non prescription oral anesthetic gel for stomatitis (painful mouth irritation) that is a common unwanted side effect of cancer chemotherapy.

**Zinecard®** *See* Dexrazoxane.

**Zithromax®** *See* Azithromycin.

**Zofran®** *See* Ondansetron.

**Zoladex®** *See* Goserelin.

**Zollinger-Ellison (ZE) syndrome** Severe, difficult-to-control ulcers of the stomach or small intestine that cause severe pain or bleeding due to increased stomach acid and sometimes cause severe diarrhea. The ZE syndrome is caused by gastrinoma, a usually malignant tumor of islet cells of the pancreas (and less often, small intestine), which may be part of the MEN syndrome. Excessive amounts of gastrin, a hormone normally found only in the stomach, cause the stomach to produce large amounts of acid. Although the majority of gastrinomas are cancer (they have spread to other sites in the abdomen), they are usually slow growing. If symptoms of stomach pain, bleeding, or diarrhea are controlled, people with ZE syndrome can lead extended, normal lives. Treatment that previously relied on total gastrectomy (removal of the entire stomach) now focuses on therapy using drugs, such as omeprazole to block production of stomach acid, together with surgery or chemotherapy to control the cancer.

℞ **Zoloft®** *See* Sertraline Hydrochloride.

℞ **zolpidem tartrate** Also known by the trade name Ambien®, this is a hypnotic (sleep inducer) drug that resembles a benzodiazepine ring. It is used to treat insomnia.

℞ **Zosyn®** *See* Piperacillin Sodium Combined with Tazobactam Sodium.

℞ **Zovirax®** *See* Acyclovir.

℞ **Zurinol®** *See* Allopurinol.

℞ **Zyban®** *See* Bupropion Hydrochloride.

℞ **Zyloprim®** *See* Allopurinol.

℞ **Zyvox®** *See* Linezolid.

# Highights on Specific Cancers

This section consists of highlights for selected cancers, such as key statistics, type of tumor and spread, risk factors, symptoms, diagnosis, determining stage, and other considerations. The statistics presented, such as the number of cases diagnosed and deaths that occur each year, are estimates based on the year of this publication. For more detailed and current information about specific cancers, please contact the American Cancer Society (ACS) at 800-ACS-2345 (www.cancer.org).

The causes of many cancers are not fully understood. However, we do know what many of the risk factors are and how some of these risk factors cause cells to become cancerous. For example, we know that many of the chemicals found in tobacco result in damage to DNA, which contains the cell's instructions for repair and growth. A risk factor is anything that increases a person's chance of getting a disease such as cancer. Different cancers have different risk factors. For example, unprotected exposure to strong sunlight is a risk factor for skin cancer; and smoking is a risk factor for cancers of the lungs, larynx, mouth, esophagus, bladder, kidneys, and several other organs.

But having a risk factor, or even several, does not mean that you will develop the disease. Many people with one or more risk factors never develop cancer, while others with this disease have no known risk factors. It is important, however, that you know about risk factors so that you can try to change any unhealthy lifestyle behaviors and choose to have the early detection tests for a potential cancer. The most commonly known risk factors are listed for each specific cancer in this section.

Only selected highlights regarding treatment considerations are included. Contact ACS for current, detailed treatment information. The choice of treatment depends on the type of cancer, location, and stage of disease, as well as age, health status, personal preferences, and other factors. Consult your doctor about your unique medical condition.

# ANAL CANCER

## Overview

The anus is the opening at the lower end of the digestive tract through which solid waste is passed. It consists of two parts: 1) the anal canal, a ¾-inch passage between the rectum and the perianal skin surrounding the anus, which is lined with mucosa continuous with that of the rectum; 2) the anal margin, the junction where the mucosa joins the hairy perianal skin. Anal lymph nodes are present in both the pelvic area and groin. Cancer of the anus is uncommon, and accounts for only a small percentage of malignancies of the digestive tract. About 3,500 cases are diagnosed each year, leading to almost 500 deaths. It occurs somewhat more often in women, but over the last 10 years it has been seen increasingly in men less than 45 years old who have acquired immunodeficiency syndrome (AIDS).

## Type of Tumor and Spread

Squamous cell carcinoma is the most common. Anal canal cancer usually metastasizes (spreads) upward to involve nodes in the pelvic area and abdomen; and anal margin cancer most often involves lymph nodes in the groin. Spread through blood to distant organs, such as the liver and lungs, occurs more often with anal canal cancer adjacent to the lower part of the rectum.

## Risk Factors

Although anal cancer occurs often in HIV-positive homosexual and bisexual men, human immunoviruses have not proven to be the cause. Human papillomavirus, which causes benign (noncancerous) warts around the anus, is thought to be the major cause of anal cancer and is related to sexual activity. Sexual activity is strongly associated with the development of anal cancer. An anal fistula, a small passage between the rectum and perianal skin due to perirectal abscess, is also associated with this cancer. Transplant patients who have their immune systems suppressed to prevent organ rejection are also at a higher risk.

## Symptoms

Slight rectal bleeding occurs in more than 50% of cancer patients. However, anal itching and burning and painful bowel movements, which are often blamed on hemorrhoids and other benign (noncancerous) conditions, may be the first indication. Painless swelling in the groin from cancer spread to the lymph node(s) may be the first symptom.

## Diagnosis

Often delayed because cancer can be confused with a hemorrhoid containing a thrombosed hemorrhoid (blood clot). Any anal sore or ulcer with a firm or hard edge felt on rectal examination is very suspicious, particularly if there are swollen lymph nodes in the groin. Anoscopy, a procedure using a lighted instrument to visualize the anus and lower rectum for examination and biopsy, is used to obtain the correct diagnosis.

### Determining Stage

A thorough physical, including careful examination of the anus and rectum, and pelvic examination in women, is done first. Needle biopsy is used to diagnose a tumor that has spread to groin lymph nodes, and a rectal sonogram is used to determine the extent of cancer around the anus. A chest x-ray and a computed tomography (CT) scan of the lower portion of the abdomen and liver are used to identify distant spread or metastasis.

### Considerations

Over the last 20 years, the use of both radiation therapy and chemotherapy has revolutionized the treatment of anal canal cancer and, in most cases, is the preferred initial treatment. Abdominoperineal resection that requires a colostomy is usually reserved for cancer that returns after combined treatment. The "ideal" therapy is unknown, and research continues to develop chemotherapy and radiation treatments that have fewer complications.

*See also* Human Papillomavirus.

## BILE DUCT CANCER

### Overview

The bile ducts convey bile from the liver into the duodenum (upper small intestine), the major portion of which is the common bile duct, a short Y-shaped tubular structure about the diameter of a large drinking straw. The ducts are made up of two layers: a soft velvety inner lining (mucosa) and a stronger outer covering. Although bile duct cancer (cholangiocarcinoma) is rare in the United States (about 3,000 cases each year), it remains a common problem in Asia and the Middle East. Bile duct cancer is usually seen in older people (over age 65) and affects slightly more men than women.

### Type of Tumor and Spread

Almost all bile duct cancers (over 95%) are adenocarcinomas that arise in the mucosal lining, most often in bile ducts above where they join to form the common duct. Spread of cancer results from tumor growth into the liver and other surrounding organs, involvement of adjacent lymph nodes, and spread through the blood to distant organs.

### Risk Factors

Persistent irritation of the ducts appears to be the major risk factor. In the United States, it is associated with cholangitis (chronic inflammatory disease of bile ducts) that sometimes occurs with chronic ulcerative colitis of the colon. The large number of these cancers in Asia and the Middle East is attributed to chronic irritation from worm-like parasites (liver flukes) in the ducts.

### Symptoms

Jaundice (yellow staining of the eyes and skin) due to obstruction of bile is first. This is usually followed by cola-colored urine and putty-colored stool as bile flow is increasingly blocked. Abdominal discomfort, fever, poor appetite, and weight loss occur as cancer progresses.

### Diagnosis

Usually suspected from CT or ultrasonography of the abdomen, but a definite diagnosis before surgery requires either biopsy using a needle directed into the tumor, or examination of the duct using endoscopy (ERCP).

### Determining Stage

A careful history taking and thorough physical examination are followed by blood tests that include liver function and blood clotting. Imaging studies include chest x-ray and abdominal CT.

### Considerations

Surgery is the main type of treatment used for bile duct cancer. However, present-day therapy seldom cures the disease, except for early cancer in the mid-portion of the duct. New methods combining radiation and chemotherapy with surgery are needed to improve results. Closer supervision of people with chronic cholangitis and inflammatory bowel disease (who are at greater risk) is needed to detect early cancers, which are more likely to be cured. Control of liver flukes should reduce the occurrence of this malignancy in the Far East.

*See also* Bile; Cholangitis; Liver Fluke.

## BLADDER CANCER

### Overview

The urinary bladder is a muscular sac-like organ in the pelvic area, which collects urine produced by the kidneys. Urine enters the bladder through the long tube-like ureter from each kidney and drains through a short passage (urethra) that in males passes through the prostate and penis. Cancer of the bladder is the most frequent malignant tumor of the urinary system (kidney, ureter, bladder, urethra) and occurs most often in older males. Whites are two times more likely to develop bladder cancer than African Americans. It is estimated that more than 54,000 Americans develop bladder cancer each year and about 12,400 die from it.

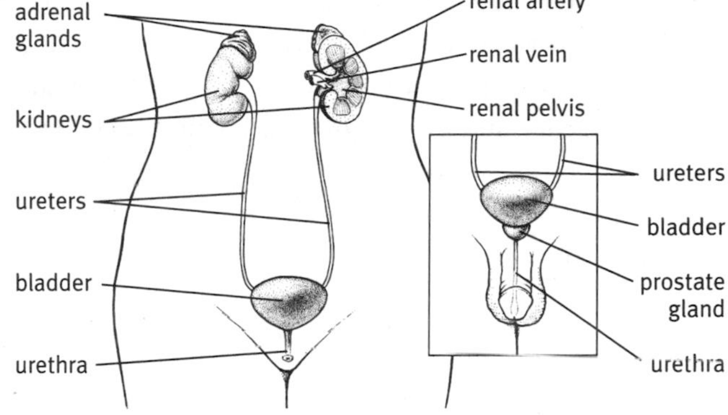


### Type of Tumor and Spread

Ninety percent of bladder cancers are urothelial carcinomas (transitional cell carcinomas) that arise in the cells that line the bladder. Urothelial tumors are divided into several subtypes according to whether they are noninvasive or invasive and whether their shape is papillary or flat.

### Risk Factors

Carcinogens (cancer-causing substances) in the urine are the most likely risk factors. Chemical workers in the aniline dye industry are especially at risk, and cigarette smokers are more than twice as likely as nonsmokers to develop the malignancy.

### Symptoms

Changes in bladder habits and/or hematuria (blood in urine) that are painless and often intermittent are usually the first complaints. Frequent, difficult, or painful urination occurs as cancer progresses.

### Diagnosis

Often, there are few findings other than bloody urine. In advanced-stage cancer, a lump or mass may be felt on rectal examination. Finding cancer cells in a urine specimen sometimes provides the diagnosis, but biopsy of the interior of the bladder using cystoscopy is usually necessary.

### Determining Stage

Examination of the interior of the bladder using a cystoscope under general or a spinal anesthetic is necessary in every case. Imaging studies include chest x-ray, bone scan, and CT or MRI of the pelvic area. Blood tests to evaluate kidney function are also needed.

### Considerations

Early disease is treated with resection of tumors through the cystoscope and with instillation of chemotherapy or, most commonly, BCG. In more advanced disease, radiation therapy and cystectomy are used, although they are often unable to control the cancer; chemotherapy only slows metastasis (spread). New methods combining drugs, hormones, and radiation with surgery are being investigated to improve results without the need for cystectomy. Investigation continues to improve the artificial bladder.

## BONE CANCER

### Overview

Cancer that originates in bone (primary cancer) is unusual and is much less common than cancer spread to the bone from other malignancies, especially prostate and breast. Fewer than 3,000 cases of bone cancer are diagnosed each year, leading to about 1,400 deaths. Primary bone cancer receives a great deal of attention because it commonly occurs in children who may require amputation of an arm or leg. Nonwhite boys and girls are less likely to be affected than are young white males. Today, more than 50% of those who develop primary bone cancer live for 5 or more years following treatment, and amputation is not always necessary.

### Type of Tumor and Spread

All primary bone cancers are sarcomas that include *osteogenic sarcoma* (osteosarcoma), which occurs most often in the knee, thigh, or arm; *chondrosarcoma,* a cancer of cells that produce cartilage (firm rubbery tissue in joints), which occurs most often in the pelvis, leg, or shoulder, in older adults; and *Ewing's sarcoma,* which develops from primitive nerve-like cells in bone marrow, which occurs most often in the leg, arm, or pelvis. There are also several other rare types of bone cancer. Distant spread from primary bone cancer is most often to the lung.

### Risk Factors

Evidence suggests a defective gene in some cases. Children with inherited neuroblastoma are more likely to develop osteosarcoma, as are children previously treated with radiation therapy or alkylating-types of chemotherapy drugs for unrelated malignancies. Adults with Paget's disease, a benign (noncancerous) bone condition, are at greater risk for osteosarcoma.

### Symptoms

Anyone, especially a child, without previous injury, who has persistent pain or a lump deep in an arm or a leg, is suspect. Furthermore, loss of bladder or bowel control indicates cancer in the lower spine involving the spinal cord or spinal nerves. Minor injury can cause pathologic fracture (a break in bone weakened by tumor). Ewing's sarcoma can cause generalized symptoms such as poor appetite, weight loss, chills and fever, and malaise (feeling poorly).

### Diagnosis

To distinguish cancer from a benign growth, a biopsy is necessary, which must be done carefully to prevent the spread of cancer cells that could interfere with future surgery. Although needle biopsy may be sufficient for diagnosis, incisional biopsy that provides a larger tissue specimen is usually needed.

### Determining Stage

A thorough history taking and physical examination are followed by x-rays, CT, and possibly MRI of the involved area, which is then followed by a bone scan. Chest x-ray and chest CT are also needed. Blood tests include liver function studies.

### Considerations

Chemotherapy with multiple drugs has greatly increased life expectancy for most types of cancer. Chemotherapy can usually shrink the cancer before surgery and has enabled limb-sparing procedures, in many instances, to give results equal to amputation. Research continues to devise treatment methods that will improve results while shortening the time needed to complete therapy.

*See also* Childhood Cancer; Ewing's Sarcoma; Paget's Disease.

## BRAIN TUMOR

### Overview

The brain and spinal cord make up the central nervous system (CNS), the site of tumors that arise inside the skull and spinal column as well as those spread from other cancers. However, the term "brain tumor" is used to describe only those originating within the skull, called primary brain cancers, rather than those that have metastasized (spread) to the brain from other parts of the body. They most often affect two age groups: children and older adults (average age = 70 years). It is estimated that approximately 17,200 Americans develop CNS tumors each year and about 13,100 die from them. For unknown reasons, primary brain tumors are becoming more common in all age groups and are second only to acute leukemia as the leading cause of cancer deaths in American children. Metastatic cancer to the central nervous system results from advanced-stage malignancies that usually are fatal.

### Type of Tumor and Spread

Central nervous system tumors of adults and children often form in different areas and from different cell types and may have a different prognosis and treatment. Although some tumors grow so slowly as to be considered benign, nearly all that originate in the brain may prove fatal unless removed. They are divided into two broad categories: gliomas and nongliomas. The former arises in glial cells that support neurons, which are the cells responsible for brain function. Although some gliomas develop slowly, many are glioblastoma multiforme that grow rapidly and always recur following treatment. All gliomas can cause death. Among tumors classified as gliomas are astrocytomas, oligodendrogliomas, and ependymomas. Nongliomas are a diverse group of tumors, which include meningiomas that arise in the meninges (covering of the brain) and are rarely malignant; medulloblastomas; primitive neuroectodermal tumors; nerve tumors, including acoustic neuromas, optic neuromas, neurofibromas—all of which are seldom malignant; craniopharyngioma; and pituitary tumors.

### Risk Factors

The large majority of brain cancers are not associated with any risk factors. Brain lymphoma, however, is associated with HIV infection.

### Symptoms

All CNS tumors cause symptoms either from growing into and destroying nerve tissue or from increasing pressure within the skull or spine. Symptoms vary widely, depending on tumor location and size. Headache, seizures, gradual paralysis, and personality change are common symptoms. Other symptoms include change in senses (sight, hearing, smell, touch, taste); nausea, vomiting, weakness; difficulty in speaking or walking; and mental deterioration, resulting from destruction of central nervous tissue. Difficulty with bladder or bowel control occurs from tumors involving the spinal cord.

### Diagnosis

Findings on physical examination of the nervous system (neurological examination) usually indicate a tumor's location, and CT and MRI are imaging studies that identify the exact site. MRI can sometimes help determine tumor type (glioblastoma multiforme), but biopsy is usually necessary to identify the growth. In cases where surgical removal is not planned, needle biopsy through a burr hole (small opening) in the skull is used to accurately diagnose the tumor. In cases of metastatic cancer, detailed laboratory and x-ray studies are often necessary to determine tumor origin and other sites of spread.

### Determining Stage

There currently is no staging system for brain tumors. The most important factors in determining outcome are cell type (astrocytoma) and grade (aggressiveness of the tumor cells).

### Considerations

Although the outlook for most malignant brain tumors is poor, surgery, rad tion, and chemotherapy can prolong and improve the lives of many patier The prognosis for children with brain tumors tends to be more favorak Because the blood-brain barrier prevents most chemotherapy from entering the CNS, newer methods of drug delivery are needed to enable anticancer drugs to pass from the blood into brain tissue.

## BREAST CANCER

### Overview

The growth and development of the breasts are influenced by estrogen, the primary female hormone produced in the ovaries. During pregnancy, mammary (breast) tissue enlarges in preparation for nursing. In males, breast tissue remains in an immature, child-like state. Although breast cancer is uncommon in young women, it is becoming more prevalent in older females. It affects approximately 10% to 11% of American women, and the number of women who survive has increased over the last decade. It is estimated that approximately 192,200 American women develop breast cancer each year and about 40,200 die from it. African Americans are more likely to die from this cancer because they are often diagnosed at an advanced stage when breast cancer is harder to treat and cure and because the cancer is often more aggressive. Although male breast cancer is rare, with only 1,500 cases estimated each year, 400 men (27%) die from the disease. For both men and women, the likelihood of survival decreases as cancer involves the axillary (underarm) lymph nodes. In those without spread to lymph nodes, the possibility of survival depends mainly on the size of the cancer. Ten years after starting treatment, 80% of women without axillary lymph node metastasis and 50% of those with lymph node metastasis are alive without cancer. Nine out of ten women with a cancer ½ inch or smaller are usually cured.

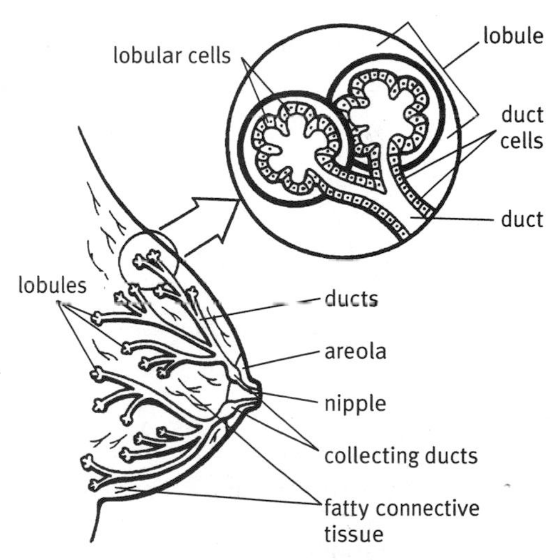


### Type of Tumor and Spread

Almost all breast cancers are adenocarcinomas that arise either in the milk-producing lobules (glands) or, more commonly, in the ducts through which milk flows to the nipple. Early cancer within a lobule (never seen in males) is known as lobular carcinoma in situ (LCIS), and early cancer within a duct is known as ductal carcinoma in situ (DCIS). Cancer that invades (grows into) surrounding breast tissue is known as infiltrating carcinoma. Although in situ breast cancer never metastasizes, infiltrating carcinoma is prone to spread first to axillary lymph nodes and later to other organs (bone, brain, liver, ovary). Inflammatory breast cancer is a rapidly growing tumor that resembles breast infection, with heat, swelling, redness, and tenderness. Paget's disease of the breast is a condition of older women, in which an intraductal cancer beneath the nipple is associated with irritation of the nipple and areola (surrounding dark, wrinkled skin).

## Risk Factors

About 10% of women with breast cancer have an inherited form of disease due to an abnormal gene, either BRCA1 or BRCA2. Inherited mutations of the p53 tumor suppressor gene can also increase a woman's risk of developing breast cancer. It is still not clear what part oral contraceptives (birth control pills) might play in breast cancer risk. However, replacement hormones (estrogen and progesterone) taken for many years (5 or more) after menopause may slightly increase the risk. Other factors associated with an increased risk of breast cancer include alcohol use, obesity and high-fat diets, not having children, not breast feeding, early menstrual periods (before age 12), late menopause (after age 50), and previous chest area irradiation. Although we know some of the risk factors that increase a woman's chance of developing breast cancer, we do not yet know what causes most breast cancers or exactly how some of these risk factors cause cells to become cancerous.

## Symptoms

A painless breast lump is by far the most common symptom, but swelling under the arm may be the first indication. Other signs of breast cancer include skin irritation or dimpling, nipple pain or retraction (turning inward), redness or scaliness of the nipple or breast skin, or a discharge other than breast milk. In men, a lump beneath the nipple is usually the first symptom noted.

## Diagnosis

A diagnostic mammogram (x-ray examination of the breast) is used for women who have a breast problem (for example, a breast mass, nipple discharge, etc.) or who have an abnormality that was found on a screening mammogram. In some cases, special images (cone views with magnification) are used to make a small area of altered breast tissue easier to evaluate. A negative mammogram, however, does not mean there is no cancer. Biopsy may be done by using a needle directed into a lump, or by surgically removing all or part of the mass. Other techniques using large needles (core needle), directed by x-ray or sonography, enable samples to be taken from small tumors and suspicious areas that in the past had to be removed completely.

**Determining Stage**

After a thorough medical examination, liver function studies and imaging studies, such as chest x-rays and bone and liver scans, may be obtained if they are indicated.

**Considerations**

Removal of the primary tumor is necessary to cure breast cancer; however, the choice of treatment (surgery, chemotherapy, hormonal manipulation) depends on the type of tumor, location, and stage of disease, as well as age, health status, personal preferences, and other factors. More women's lives can be saved in the future if more women and health care professionals take advantage of early detection tests (mammograms, clinical breast exams, breast self-exams). Following screening guidelines can improve chances of survival by finding breast cancer early when it is highly curable (*see* Appendix for Cancer Detection Guidelines). Much research is currently being done on a variety of risk factors (BRCA gene, lifestyle habits), chemoprevention methods (tamoxifen), and improved treatment techniques (sentinel node procedure).

*See also* Biopsy; BRCA; Breast Conservation Therapy; Breast Implant; Breast Reconstruction Surgery; CA 15-3; DCIS; HER2/*neu*; Lumpectomy; Mammogram; Mammography; Mammoplasty; Mastectomy; Paget's Disease.

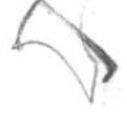

# CERVICAL CANCER

**Overview**

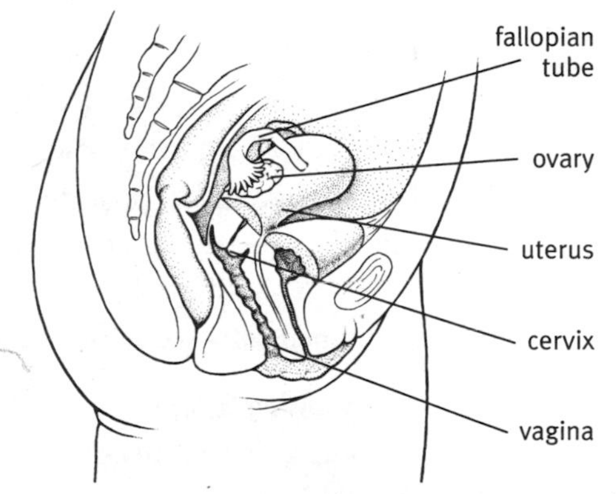


The uterine cervix is the elongated lower part (neck) of the womb where it joins the upper part of the birth canal (vagina). Although cervical cancer remains a common malignancy, today it is much less of a threat because the Pap (Papanicolaou) test makes it possible to detect and cure early disease. Once the most common malignancy of female reproductive organs, cervical cancer now occurs less often than ovarian and endometrial cancers. It is estimated that almost 13,000 American women develop cervical cancer each year and approximately 4,400 die from it. Several racial and ethnic groups (African Americans, Hispanics, and Native Americans) have cervical cancer death rates that are higher than the national average. Clearly, most of these deaths could be prevented if women routinely have the simple, inexpensive Pap smear.

### Type of Tumor and Spread

Squamous cell carcinoma, which first spreads to adjacent lymph nodes and later to the rectum, bladder, and other pelvic organs is the most common (85% to 90%) type. The remaining 10% to 15% of cervical cancers are adenocarcinomas, which develop from the mucus-producing gland cells of the endocervix. Spread via blood to organs outside the pelvis is unusual.

### Risk Factors

The major risk factor for cervical cancer is infection with the human papillomavirus that causes genital warts. Certain types are more likely to be associated with cervical cancer than others. The virus is transmitted by sexual contact so that starting sexual activity early in life and having many partners are risk factors. HIV infection is also a risk factor. Smokers are about twice as likely as nonsmokers to develop cervical cancer. Although full blown cervical cancers don't usually begin till women are in their 30s or older, a very early form, carcinoma in situ, occurs in women 10 to 25 years younger.

### Symptoms

Early cervical cancer usually shows no symptoms. Clear or bloody vaginal discharge, especially following intercourse, is often the first indication. Later, increased bleeding and aching in the pelvic area or rectum may occur. Low back pain, difficulty urinating or moving the bowels, and blood in the stool or urine indicate advanced cancer.

### Diagnosis

A reddening or growth on the cervix seen on a pelvic examination is very suggestive, although early cancer (carcinoma in situ) may show little or no change. Pap smear usually provides the correct diagnosis; but cervical biopsy, using a lighted magnifying instrument (colposcope), may be needed. Conization, in which a cone-shaped piece of tissue is taken from the cervix for biopsy, is necessary when colposcopy is inadequate for diagnosis.

### Determining Stage

A comprehensive history taking and careful physical examination are usually followed by a more extensive pelvic examination under general anesthesia. Blood tests to evaluate kidney and liver function may be needed. Imaging studies include chest x-ray and, in many cases, CT of the lower abdomen and pelvis. Cystoscopy to view the bladder and sigmoidoscopy to examine the rectum may also be advised.

### Considerations

Following screening guidelines for Pap tests and pelvic examinations can improve the chances of successful treatment by finding cervical cancer early when it is highly curable (*see* Appendix for Cancer Detection Guidelines). The Pap test can find precancerous changes called cervical intraepithelial neoplasia (CIN) that can be treated to prevent them from progressing to a cancer. Today, as women begin sexual activity at an early age and with multiple partners, the number of young females with very early cancers, such as carcinoma in situ, will likely increase. Control of in situ cervical cancer probably will depend on controlling sexually transmitted viral diseases. Much research is currently being done to find new ways to prevent and treat cervical cancer (oncogenes, tumor suppressor genes, HPV tests).

*See also* Human Papillomavirus; Hysterectomy; Pap Test; Pelvic Examination.

## COLORECTAL CANCER

### Overview

The large intestine (bowel) is the lower portion of the tube-like intestinal tract, whose function is to absorb water from intestinal contents and store and eliminate feces (solid waste). It is arbitrarily divided into two parts: the colon and rectum. The colon is the upper or proximal part (about 6 feet long) that lies entirely within the abdomen. It begins at the termination of the small intestine and ends at the rectum. The rectum is the last 8 inches of the large bowel in the pelvis below the abdomen, which terminates at the anus. The colon consists of five parts: cecum, right or ascending colon, transverse colon, left (descending) colon, and sigmoid colon. Colorectal cancer is the fourth most common cancer found in the United States (excluding skin cancers). It is estimated that approximately 135,400 men and women, usually over 50 years of age, develop this malignancy each year and about 56,700 die from it.

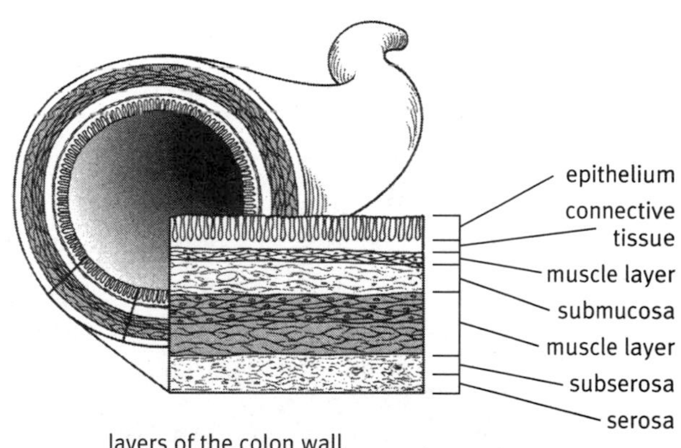

layers of the colon wall

### Type of Tumor and Spread

Adenocarcinoma of the mucosa (lining) of the large intestine is the most common (95%) type. Cancer of the right colon (i.e., cecum, ascending colon, first 14 inches of transverse colon) usually forms a heaped-up cauliflower-like growth that bleeds easily, while cancer in the left colon (i.e., last 14 inches of the transverse colon, descending colon, and sigmoid colon) and rectum characteristically forms a firm tumor that narrows and often blocks or obstructs the intestine. With time, tumors grow through the mucosa to involve the underlying muscle layer and later penetrate through the bowel wall. Metastasis (spread) outside the intestine is first to the lymph nodes and then through the blood to distant organs, especially the liver and lung. Metastasis within the abdomen or peritoneal cavity results from cancer involving adjacent organs or malignant cells shed throughout the abdominal cavity.

## Risk Factors

Most cancers arise as adenomatous polyps (mushroom-like growths) in the mucosa (lining), and the likelihood of cancer increases as the polyps grow in size. In familial adenomatous polyposis (FAP), an inherited condition in which thousands of polyps carpet the mucosa, cancer develops in every case, unless the involved intestine is removed at an early age. Another inherited condition, hereditary nonpolyposis colon cancer (HNPCC), occurs in family members without large numbers of polyps. People with inflammatory bowel diseases (chronic ulcerative colitis, Crohn's disease of the colon) that begin at an early age are at increased risk. Diet, particularly one high in fat, may lead to polyps that progress to cancer. People who are obese, physically inactive, or smoke are at increased risk of developing the disease. Cigarette smoking is estimated to cause almost 12% of fatal colorectal cancers and smokers are 30% to 40% more likely to die of colorectal cancer than nonsmokers.

## Symptoms

A change in usual bowel habits, either constipation or diarrhea, is often the first indication; and narrowing of the stool may occur with rectal tumors. Rectal bleeding may be noticed in cancers of the rectum and descending (left) colon, but unrecognized bleeding that causes anemia (low number of red blood cells), with weakness, fatigue, and pale skin, often occurs with tumors of the ascending (right) colon. Both cramping abdominal pain and rectal discomfort indicate more advanced-stage disease, as does abdominal swelling due to either intestinal blockage or fluid buildup.

## Diagnosis

Any growth in the colon or rectum is very suspicious, and cancer usually presents a characteristic picture on barium enema and colonoscopy. However, biopsy obtained during colonoscopy is necessary for the diagnosis.

### Determining Stage

A careful history taking and physical examination, with particular attention to abdominal and rectal findings, is followed by blood tests that include complete blood count (CBC), liver function, and the tumor marker carcinoembryonic antigen (CEA). Imaging studies include chest x-ray and abdominal CT. Rectal endoscopic ultrasonography (EUS) is very useful for evaluating the depth of invasion and for identifying enlarged adjacent lymph nodes in rectal cancer.

### Considerations

Following screening guidelines can lower the number of cases of the disease by detecting and removing polyps that could become cancerous and can also lower the death rate from colorectal cancer by finding disease early when it is highly curable (*see* Appendix for Cancer Detection Guidelines). Prevention and early detection are possible because most colon cancers develop from adenomatous polyps. Polyps are precancerous growths in the colon and rectum. Removing them can lower a person's risk by preventing some colorectal cancers before they are fully formed.

Celecoxib (Celebrex®) used to treat arthritis has been approved for people with familial adenomatous polyposis to cut down on the number of colorectal polyps and the risk of cancer. People can also lower their risk of developing colorectal cancer by managing the risk factors that they can control, such as diet and physical activity. Because today's methods to examine the colon and rectum can be somewhat unpleasant and uncomfortable, less cumbersome methods to diagnose polyps and early cancers are being studied, but not yet recommended for routine use. However, colonoscopy, double contrast barium enema, flexible sigmoidoscopy, and the fecal occult blood test are tools for the present to reduce deaths from colorectal cancers.

*See also* Colectomy; Colon; Colonoscope; Colonoscopy; Small Intestine Cancer (pages 201–202).

## ENDOMETRIAL CANCER

### Overview

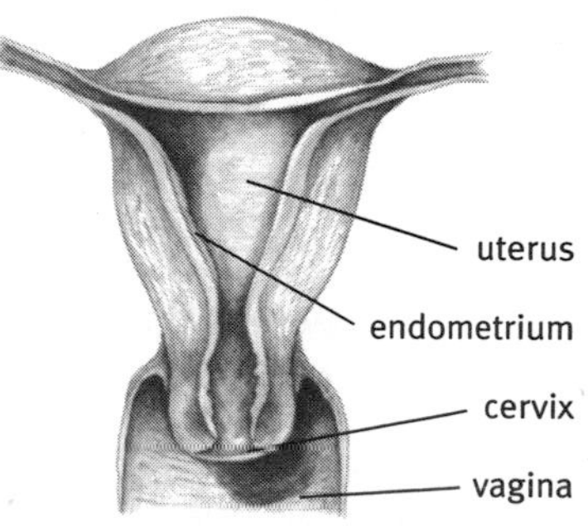


The endometrium is the lining of the womb or uterus where an egg fertilized in a fallopian tube attaches and develops into an embryo. In women of childbearing age, each month the endometrium, in response to hormones from the ovaries, thickens with new blood vessels for possible pregnancy. If fertilization does not take place, then the endometrium is shed through menstruation, after which the cycle is repeated.

Cancer of the endometrium, the most common malignancy of female reproductive organs, is seen most often in older women past menopause, with 95% of cases occurring after age 40. It is estimated that about 38,300 American women develop this cancer each year and approximately 6,600 die of it. Treated at an early stage, endometrial cancer is almost always curable.

## Type of Tumor and Spread

Adenocarcinoma, the most common variety, spreads over the surface of the endometrium before growing deeper into, or invading, the underlying uterine muscle. Metastasis (spread of cancer) can occur from cancer cells spreading through the fallopian tubes into the abdomen, via lymphatics to adjacent or regional lymph nodes, and in blood to distant organs, such as the lung, bone, and liver.

## Risk Factors

Uninterrupted growth of the endometrium appears to be the most likely risk factor—either from prolonged estrogen secretion by the ovaries, as in delayed menopause, or from estrogen replacement therapy for menopausal women. Women who are obese, eat high-fat diets, have few, if any, children, and start menopause at a late age are at greater risk. Tamoxifen, used to treat or prevent breast cancer, can also cause this cancer. Young women who do not receive replacement estrogen following bilateral oophorectomy (removal of both ovaries), as well as those who take birth control pills are less likely to develop endometrial cancer.

## Symptoms

In a woman past menopause, vaginal discharge of any kind, especially containing blood, is often the first indication of endometrial cancer. Younger women may notice irregular or prolonged menstrual periods.

## Diagnosis

An enlarged uterus or a mass is sometimes felt on pelvic examination, but the pelvic examination result is often normal, especially in the early stages. Endometrial biopsy, which is often done in physicians' offices without anesthesia, usually provides the correct diagnosis. However, a minor operation under general anesthesia to scrape out the endometrium (dilatation and curettage or D&C) may be needed. A Pap test is helpful in diagnosing endometrial cancer in only 20% of cases.

## Determining Stage

A thorough physical examination that includes careful pelvic and rectal examination is followed by blood studies to evaluate kidney and liver function. Imaging studies include chest x-ray and CT of the abdomen and pelvis. In advanced cancer, cystoscopy and sigmoidoscopy may be needed to identify involvement of bladder and rectum.

### Considerations

Although uterine cancer is curable in most cases, over the past 30 years there has been little increase in the number of women cured. Newer methods using both radiation therapy and drugs are needed as the population of older women increases and as cervical cancer becomes more common. The American Cancer Society includes endometrial biopsy in its recommendations for early detection of cancer in certain women (*see* Appendix for Cancer Detection Guidelines).

*See also* Pap Test; Pelvic Examination.

## ESOPHAGEAL CANCER

### Overview

The esophagus is the muscular tube that connects the throat and stomach. It is about 10 inches long and is lined with squamous epithelium. The upper 2 inches are in the neck behind the windpipe or trachea, and the remainder lies in the middle of the chest (mediastinum). In the United States, esophageal cancer occurs three times more often in men, especially in African Americans. In parts of some countries, such as China and Iran, the incidence of esophageal cancer is 30 to 40 times that in the US. It is estimated that about 13,200 Americans develop esophageal cancer each year and approximately 12,500 die of it.

### Type of Tumor and Spread

Cancer arises in the mucosal lining, and in the past, 90% of these cancers were squamous cell carcinomas. However, over the past 3 decades, there has been a marked increase in the number of cases of adenocarcinoma of the lower esophagus adjacent to the stomach (gastrointestinal junction); these now account for almost 50% of all esophageal malignant tumors. Cancer disseminates either by growing beneath the mucosa (inner lining), by involving adjacent organs, or by spreading to lymph nodes and distant organs, most often the liver and lungs. Dysplasia (precancerous change) in the mucosal lining of the esophagus often precedes actual cancer.

### Risk Factors

In the United States, cigarette smoking associated with heavy alcohol consumption appears to be responsible for most cases of squamous cell carcinoma. Barrett's esophagus, in which the usual squamous cells lining the esophagus change to columnar cells that are normally found in the stomach, is a know precursor of adenocarcinoma. Plummer-Vinson syndrome, an esophageal condition resulting from a deficiency of vitamins and iron, is associated with esophageal cancer, especially in Scandinavian women. Also, people with head and neck cancer are 10 times more likely to develop esophageal squamous carcinoma.

### Symptoms

Difficulty swallowing food, most often bread or meat, is the first indication, which varies from slight chest discomfort to food sticking in the throat. About 50% of patients experience weight loss. Later symptoms include hoarseness, hiccups, difficulty swallowing liquids, and burning or cramping in the chest. Inability to swallow saliva indicates complete obstruction by a tumor.

### Diagnosis

Few, if any, physical findings are usual. Obvious weight loss, enlarged lymph nodes in the neck, and hoarseness are found only after cancer progresses. Although findings on barium swallow are very suggestive, biopsy obtained by esophagoscopy (a type of endoscopy) is necessary for the correct diagnosis.

### Determining Stage

A thorough physical examination is followed by blood tests that determine liver function as well as a chest x-ray and CT. Endoscopic ultrasonography of the esophagus (EUS) provides the most accurate evaluation of tumor thickness. Bronchoscopy is necessary in cancer of the upper esophagus to determine whether the adjacent trachea (windpipe) is involved. A newer test, the PET scan, provides a good estimate of whether the cancer has spread to the lymph nodes.

### Considerations

Although the outlook for this malignancy is poor, improved surgical techniques combined with new methods of drug therapy and radiation therapy are likely to make future treatment of esophageal cancer more successful. Several studies have found that regular aspirin use reduced the likelihood of developing esophageal carcinoma by about 50%. Additional research is needed to determine whether aspirin or similar drugs should be recommended for people at increased risk for developing this cancer.

*See also* Barrett's Esophagus; Esophagoscope; Esophagoscopy; Esophagus; Head and Neck Cancer (pages 170–172); Plummer-Vinson Syndrome.

## GALLBLADDER CANCER

### Overview

The gallbladder is the small sac-like organ on the undersurface of the liver, whose function is to store and concentrate bile. Bile enters and exits through the cystic duct connected to the common bile duct that conveys bile from the liver to the intestines. Food emptying from the stomach into the duodenum (upper small intestine) causes the release of the hormone cholecystokinin, which causes the gallbladder to squeeze bile back into the common duct where it flows into the small intestine and aids in digesting fat.

Gallbladder cancer, the fifth most common cancer of the gastrointestinal tract, is found in less than 1% of operations for gallstones. Each year approximately 6,000 to 7,000 cases are diagnosed in the United States. Only 10% of all patients survive 5 years after diagnosis because it is usually discovered at an advanced stage. It remains a very lethal cancer of older people (usually over age 70), especially women. Gallbladder cancer is more common among white women than among African-American women, and it is more common among Mexican Americans and Native Americans than among the general population.

### Type of Tumor and Spread

Most gallbladder cancers (over 80%) are adenocarcinoma of the gallbladder mucosa (lining). Metastasis (spread) occurs early to both the liver and the adjacent (regional) lymph nodes.

### Risk Factors

Persistent irritation, most often due to gallstones (present in 75% to 90% of gallbladder cancers), appears to be the most likely risk factor. However, people with calcium deposits in the wall of the gallbladder (porcelain gallbladder) appear especially prone, with about 20% developing cancer. Cigarette smoking and obesity are also associated with an increased risk of the disease.

### Symptoms

At first, cancer symptoms are similar to those from gallstones and include mild discomfort in the right upper part of the abdomen in the area of the liver, slight nausea, and/or indigestion. Persistent abdominal pain and jaundice (yellow staining of eyes and skin) indicate advanced disease.

### Diagnosis

Although gallbladder ultrasonography and CT can suggest cancer prior to surgery, most early tumors are not discovered until the gallbladder is removed (cholecystectomy) for gallstones.

### Determining Stage

A thorough history taking and complete physical examination are followed by blood tests, including liver function studies. Imaging studies include a chest x-ray and CT of the abdomen.

### Considerations

Surgery offers the only hope for curing people with gallbladder cancer. As a rule, the only patients cured of this malignant tumor are those whose very small tumors are found incidentally when the gallbladder is removed for gallstones. Removing a diseased gallbladder when stones are first diagnosed can prevent gallbladder cancer.

*See also* Bile.

## HEAD AND NECK CANCER (excluding lip and larynx)

### Overview

This cancer of the aerodigestive tract (the part of the body concerned with both breathing and swallowing) includes a variety of malignant tumors of the mouth, nose, sinuses, and throat. Although these cancers are often grouped together, they differ markedly in their tendency to spread and their response to treatment. Cancer of the head and neck is fairly common and affects men almost three times as often as women, although this ratio seems to be decreasing. Approximately 30,100 new cases are diagnosed each year, leading to about 7,800 deaths. Most cancers continue to occur in older people; but due to the recent widespread use of smokeless tobacco, they are becoming more common in young men. Head and neck cancer is much more common in Hungary and France than in the United States and is less common in Mexico and Japan.

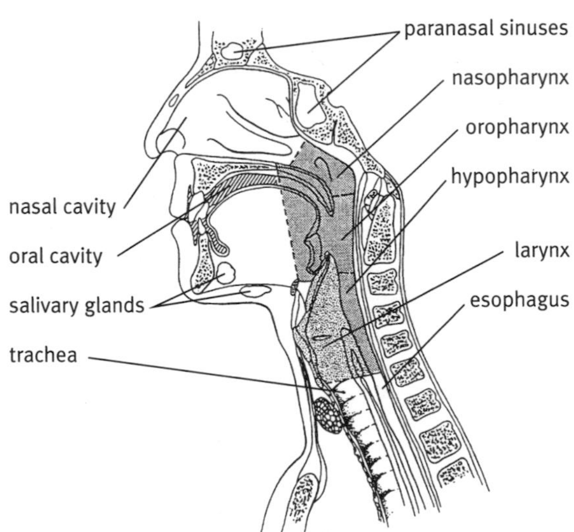


### Type of Tumor and Spread

Except for nasopharyngeal cancer, an undifferentiated variety of carcinoma, more than 90% are squamous cell carcinomas that involve the mucosa (lining) continuous throughout the head and neck region. Some cancers appear to progress from white or red, thickened precancerous areas called leukoplakia and erythroplakia, respectively, to carcinoma in situ, and later to full-blown cancer. All can grow into, or invade, bone and other tissues. Spread to cervical nodes, which are lymph node(s) in the neck, depends on the location of the original, or primary, growth. Spread outside the neck occurs late in the disease, after the cervical nodes are involved with cancer.

### Risk Factors

Abuse of both alcohol and tobacco, especially the smokeless variety (snuff), is associated with cancers of the floor of the mouth, tongue, and gum. People who smoke and drink alcohol are six times more likely to develop these cancers than those who do not. The Epstein-Barr virus (EBV) is associated with nasopharyngeal cancer. Textile, furniture, and chemical workers are prone to develop malignancies of the nose and sinuses, and people with previous head and neck cancer are much more likely to develop second, unrelated aerodigestive malignancies.

### Symptoms

Cancer of the mouth and throat usually presents as a nonhealing, painful sore and as a malignant tumor in the nose and sinus that causes breathing difficulty, nosebleed, and/or sinus pain. Painless swelling in the neck, from involved lymph node(s), may be the first indication. Other indications include difficulty chewing, swallowing, or moving the jaw or tongue; persistent lump or thickening in the cheek; and a persistent white or red patch on the gums, tongue, tonsil, or lining of the mouth.

### Diagnosis

Biopsy is usually possible under local anesthesia. Biopsy of areas other than the mouth usually requires a lighted instrument (endoscope). Cancer in the lymph nodes may be diagnosed by needle biopsy.

### Determining Stage

Following a thorough physical examination, with particular attention paid to the head and neck, a detailed examination of the nose and throat with an endoscope is necessary. Imaging studies include chest x-ray, CT or MRI of the head and neck, and barium swallow.

### Considerations

Treatment combining radiation therapy and chemotherapy prior to surgery often enables smaller operations to give the same results as more extensive surgery, without many of the unwanted postoperative problems associated with more radical operations. In advanced-stage cancers, new treatment is needed to improve the likelihood of cure while reducing unwanted side effects. Beta carotene and other chemical compounds similar to vitamin A may prevent leukoplakia (precancerous lesions) from progressing to cancer. Public awareness of the dangers of cigarettes and snuff hopefully will lead to a decrease in the occurrence of head and neck cancer. The American Cancer Society includes examination of the oral cavity in its recommendations for routine cancer-related checkups (see Appendix for Cancer Detection Guidelines).

*See also* Epstein-Barr Virus; Esophageal Cancer (pages 167–168); Laryngeal Cancer (pages 175–176); Salivary Gland Cancer (pages 198–199).

## HODGKIN'S DISEASE

### Overview

This type of lymphatic cancer usually arises in the lymph node(s), which are bean-shaped bodies up to an inch in diameter adjacent to blood vessels and are part of the body's immune (protective) mechanism. Hodgkin's disease affects almost 7,400 Americans each year, leading to about 1,300 deaths. It usually occurs in two age groups: early adulthood (ages 15–40) and late adulthood (after age 75). The disease is slightly more common in males, and the risk of developing it in the United States often parallels the individual's educational level. Treatment for most cases of Hodgkin's disease is very effective, with a 5-year survival rate close to 90% for patients under age 65.

### Type of Tumor and Spread

Hodgkin's disease differs from other (non-Hodgkin's) lymphomas by having distinctive cells called Reed-Sternberg cells in lymph nodes examined under the microscope. It is often classified into five subtypes (nodular sclerosis, mixed cellularity, lymphocyte predominant, lymphocyte depletion, unclassified) according to microscopic appearance, which sometimes helps define treatment and predict prognosis (outcome). The malignancy appears to spread first from one lymph node group to another, then to the spleen, and later to other organs.

### Risk Factors

Unlike many other types of cancer, Hodgkin's disease does not seem to be caused by a genetic disorder, diet, or the environment. Viral infection has long been suspected, especially from the Epstein-Barr virus that causes mononucleosis, an illness of younger people, with fever, sore throat, enlarged lymph nodes and spleen. However, there is no evidence of a previous Epstein-Barr virus infection in half of the patients with Hodgkin's disease; thus, its role is unclear.

### Symptoms

There are few indications of disease. Most people who have Hodgkin's disease have swollen lymph nodes that are usually painless. Sometimes the disease causes shortness of breath or coughing, fever, night sweats, tiredness, and weight loss.

### Diagnosis

Biopsy of involved lymph node(s), including the capsule (outer part) of the node, is necessary to diagnose Hodgkin's disease. Although needle biopsy does not provide enough tissue from lymph nodes to make an accurate initial diagnosis, it can identify the presence or absence of discasc in the bone marrow.

### Determining Stage

A detailed history and careful physical examination precede laboratory studies. Blood tests include a complete blood count as well as kidney and liver function tests. Imaging studies include chest x-rays, CT of the chest and abdomen. Surgery (staging laparotomy) to biopsy the liver and abdominal lymph nodes and remove the spleen was often performed in the past, however it is now rarely recommended.

### Considerations

Treatment of Hodgkin's disease has been extremely successful and represents one of medicine's greatest advances. Almost 90% of people diagnosed with Hodgkin's disease are cured with chemotherapy that is often combined with radiation therapy. Research continues for safer and more effective means of controlling this cancer. Immunotherapy may improve the possibility of curing an aggressive form of Hodgkin's disease that spreads rapidly.

*See also* Epstein-Barr Virus.

## KIDNEY CANCER

### Overview

The kidneys are paired organs that produce urine, and they are located on each side of the lower spine in the retroperitoneum, which is the area behind the abdominal cavity. Each consists of two parts: the outer portion in which urine is produced, and the renal pelvis, the collecting system in which urine is channeled into the ureter and conveyed to the bladder. The kidneys also produce erythropoietin, a hormone that enhances the formation of red blood cells. Attached to the upper pole (upper part) of each kidney is the adrenal gland, a small gland that produces several hormones, including cortisol, aldosterone, and epinephrine. Each kidney and adjacent adrenal is enclosed in a tough layer of tissue called Gerota's fascia. Renal cell carcinoma (cancer of the kidney) occurs most often between the ages of 50 and 70, and men are twice as likely to develop the tumor. It is estimated that almost 31,000 Americans (adults and children) develop kidney cancer each year and approximately 12,100 dic of it.

### Type of Tumor and Spread

Ninety percent of kidney cancers are renal cell carcinomas (hypernephromas) that arise in the urine-producing cells, and most of the remaining are transitional cell carcinomas, which begin in the renal pelvis. Wilms' tumor is an uncommon cancer of infants and young children. Renal cell cancer often involves the inferior vena cava, the large vein that drains blood from the lower body, which results in early metastasis (spread) to the lungs and other organs.

### Risk Factors

Environmental factors and chronic (persistent) kidney disease are both implicated as risk factors. Cigarette smoking increases the risk of developing renal cell carcinoma by 30% to 100%. Workers in the aniline dye industry, and possibly those in petroleum refining, are at an increased risk. Phenacetin, once widely prescribed as a pain reliever, has been linked to renal cell cancer, although this medication has not been available in the United States in over 20 years. End-stage kidney disease that requires dialysis with the artificial kidney makes people more at risk for developing this cancer. Renal cell cancer is known to occur repeatedly in some families.

### Symptoms

There are few indications until cancer is in an advanced stage, when it causes three common symptoms: pain in the lower back, bloody urine, and a lump or mass in the side below the ribs. Some individuals develop paraneoplastic syndrome (symptoms that appear to have nothing to do with the cancer), which include marked weight loss, fatigue, fever, and polycythemia (increased numbers of red blood cells).

### Diagnosis

A mass in the side of an individual who is experiencing both low back pain and passing blood is very suggestive. Cancer is usually confirmed with kidney x-rays (IVP) and possibly with ultrasonography.

### Determining Stage

Following a detailed history and complete physical examination, blood tests include kidney function studies, liver function studies, and complete blood count. A chest x-ray, and often, a CT and MRI of the chest and abdomen are advised.

### Considerations

The use of CT and ultrasonography to diagnose abdominal problems, such as gallbladder disease, has resulted in some renal cell cancers being discovered at a very early stage before they cause symptoms, when they are likely to be cured. The only curative treatment is surgery. Neither radiation nor chemotherapy is very effective for renal cell carcinoma. Immunotherapy is often used in advanced cancer.

*See also* Kidney Function Study; Retroperitoneum; Wilms' Tumor (pages 212–213).

# LARYNGEAL CANCER

## Overview

The larynx, or voice box, is a complex organ made up of five cartilages, several muscles, and a pair of vocal cords. It produces the voice, prevents swallowed material from entering the lungs, and enables coughing to clear air passages. It is divided into three parts: glottis (vocal cords), epiglottis (area above the cords), and subglottis (area below the cords). About 10,000 new cases of laryngeal cancer are diagnosed each year, leading to approximately 4,000 deaths. It is 50% more common among African Americans than among whites and tends to occur in older men (60 years and above) in the squamous epithelium (tissue lining the larynx), which is continuous with the lining of the throat and esophagus. Laryngeal cancer receives attention because treatment can result in total loss of the voice.

## Type of Tumor and Spread

Ninety-five percent of all laryngeal cancers are squamous cell carcinomas that spread by invading (growing into) adjacent tissue and involving lymph nodes in the neck. Although lymphatics in the larynx are abundant and complex, the spread of tumor to the lymph nodes often can be predicted from the location of the original (primary) tumor. Spread of tumor to distant organs (lung, liver) occurs late.

## Risk Factors

Tobacco and alcohol play a significant role in the development of this cancer. Cigarette smokers are five to thirty-five times more likely to develop this cancer than are nonsmokers, depending on how much they smoke. Heavy drinkers have a risk of developing laryngeal cancer two to five times that of nondrinkers.

## Symptoms

Laryngeal cancers that form on the glottis cause hoarseness, but the symptoms of those that form on the epiglottis and subglottis are much more vague. Sometimes problems include difficulty swallowing, sore throat, coughing, ear pain, and difficulty breathing.

## Diagnosis

Laryngeal cancer should be suspected in anyone, especially a smoker, with either persistent hoarseness or enlarged lymph node(s) in the neck. Biopsy of the tumor is usually possible using a lighted instrument passed down the throat (laryngoscopy) under local anesthesia. Needle biopsy is used to diagnose cancer that has spread to lymph node(s) in the neck.

### Determining Stage

Following laryngoscopy, a detailed history taking is followed by physical examination, with particular attention paid to the head and neck. Blood tests that include CBC and liver function are followed by an x-ray and CT of the chest and a CT or MRI of the neck.

### Considerations

Most laryngeal cancers are treated with surgery and radiation therapy, either alone or in combination, depending on the stage of the cancer. Varying degrees of hoarseness follow most treatment methods, and loss of voice occurs after total laryngectomy that requires permanent tracheostomy for breathing. Following total laryngectomy, either esophageal speech or tracheoesophageal puncture (TEP) can restore vocal communication without a buzzing instrument pressed against the neck. Today, chemotherapy and radiation therapy can control some advanced-stage disease without the need for sacrificing the voice, and in the future may be used to treat all stages without surgery. As the number of cigarette smokers declines, the incidence of laryngeal cancer should decrease.

*See also* Head and Neck Cancer (pages 170–172); Laryngectomy.

## LEUKEMIA

### Overview

Any one of a varied group of cancers that have in common the overgrowth of abnormal leukocytes (white blood cells) in bone marrow, blood, and internal organs. It affects 31,500 people each year, leading to 21,500 deaths. Leukemia is categorized as either acute (fast growing) or chronic (slow growing). They can cause severe symptoms that include extreme anemia and bleeding, although symptoms from the chronic forms often develop slowly. Left untreated, acute leukemia is often fatal within a few months. Chronic leukemia, which is most often seen in older adults, persists longer than one year, causes the gradual onset of anemia, and enlargement of the spleen, liver, and lymph nodes. Leukemias are among the most studied cancers, and the knowledge and experience gained from their treatment has been applied to more common malignancies.

### Type of Tumor and Spread

Both acute and chronic forms of the disease are classified on the basis of the type of white blood cell involved and usually are designated as either myelocytic (myelogenous) or lymphocytic. Both varieties are further divided into a number of subtypes including:

*Acute lymphoblastic leukemia (ALL):* Comprises 90% of childhood leukemia and is less common in older adults.

*Chronic lymphocytic leukemia (CLL):* The most common leukemia in the United States; it is a disease of older people that often progresses very slowly.

*Acute myelocytic leukemia (AML):* Occurs in children, but more often in older adults.

*Chronic myelocytic leukemia (CML):* Eventually changes to AML. It is most common in middle-aged adults and is rare in children.

All varieties of leukemia destroy bone marrow and interfere with the normal activity of white blood cells, red blood cells, and platelets, causing infection, anemia, and bleeding, respectively. Organs other than bone marrow, such as the lymph nodes, spleen, liver, testes, and the central nervous system (brain, meninges covering the brain), are often involved.

### Risk Factors

The only proven lifestyle-related risk factor for leukemia is cigarette smoking. Certain genetic conditions (Li-Fraumeni, Klinefelter's, and Down's syndromes) are associated with an increased risk of developing leukemia. Acute leukemia is more common in siblings, especially twins less than 6 years old. The occurrence of acute leukemia is markedly increased after radiation exposure, such as atomic bomb survivors, and after treatment with radiation therapy and certain chemotherapy drugs. Benzene exposure is another risk factor.

### Symptoms

The symptoms of leukemia vary according to organ(s) involved, but enlarged lymph nodes, spleen, and liver are often the first. Other problems include pale skin, weakness, fever, easy bruising, and bleeding (especially from the gums).

### Diagnosis

Although a CBC usually indicates leukemia, in some instances (aleukemic leukemia) the number of white blood cells in the blood may actually be lower than normal. A definite diagnosis requires a bone marrow aspiration and biopsy and, in many cases, depends on laboratory studies using monoclonal antibodies and flow cytometry. Other blood tests include liver function and blood clotting.

### Determining Stage

Because leukemia is a generalized disease affecting the entire body, determining the extent of disease (staging) is not necessary. Laboratory tests focus on accurately determining the type and subtype of acute leukemia. Different staging systems are used for different types of chronic leukemia. Some types do not have any staging system.

### Considerations

The dramatic change in leukemia from a universally fatal cancer to one that is sometimes curable, particularly in children, is remarkable. However, chemotherapy of acute leukemia remains very toxic and prolonged, and radiation therapy to the brain often causes permanent impairment. New drugs, such as Gleevec®, and monoclonal antibodies are being developed. Young patients who relapse after treatment are often treated with blood stem cell transplants from immunologically matched donors (allogeneic transplants). New methods of allogeneic transplants called "non-myelosuppressive" transplants that are less toxic are being studied for use in older patients.

## LIVER CANCER

### Overview

The liver is the largest internal organ in the body and it produces bile, albumen, and other proteins, takes part in sugar and carbohydrate (starch) metabolism, and rids the body of many toxic wastes. It is made up of two main divisions or lobes: a large right lobe and smaller left lobe, which are divided into smaller segments. The liver is the site of primary cancers originating in it and, more often, the location of metastases (spread) from other sites such as the colon, rectum, and breast. However, the term "liver cancer" is used to indicate cancer that originates in the liver, notably hepatocellular carcinoma and cholangiocarcinoma. About 16,200 new cases are diagnosed each year, leading to approximately 14,100 deaths. This cancer is about 10 times more common in developing countries in Asia, particularly East Asia, and in Africa. In the United States, liver cancer most often affects older men. Hepatoblastoma, an uncommon childhood liver cancer, occurs most often in children around age one.

### Type of Tumor and Spread

The most common type (over 80%) of liver cancer in the United States is hepatocellular cancer (hepatoma) involving cells that make up the liver substance. Tumor occurs either as a single (solitary) tumor or as multiple (diffuse) growths. Fibrolamellar hepatoma, a variety seen most often in women, is more easily controlled than the usual hepatoma. Cholangiocarcinoma of the liver arises in the bile ducts (bile collecting system). In the United States, it accounts for about 15% of liver cancers.

### Risk Factors

The risk of developing liver cancer is associated with the hepatitis B virus, hepatitis C virus, and chronic liver disease (cirrhosis). Most cirrhosis in the United

States is due to alcohol abuse, but elevated iron levels as well as hepatitis B and C are also major causes of cirrhosis. Most liver cancer in developing countries is related to hepatitis B infection. In tropical Africa, cirrhosis is sometimes caused by consumption of grain products and peanuts contaminated with *Aspergillus,* a fungus that produces aflatoxin, which is a known carcinogen (toxic substance known to cause cancer). Cholangiocarcinoma throughout Asia is often associated with parasites (liver flukes), which invade the bile ducts; and in the United States, it is sometimes related to stones in the ducts of the liver.

## Symptoms

Abdominal pain and swelling, poor appetite, and weight loss are commonly associated with hepatocellular cancer; and hypoglycemia (decreased blood sugar) that causes weakness, sweating, and fainting is the most common paraneoplastic syndrome associated with this malignancy. Jaundice (yellow staining of eyes and skin) is often the first symptom of liver cancer.

## Diagnosis

In anyone with cirrhosis, increasing jaundice or an enlarging mass in the upper right part of the abdomen is very suggestive of liver cancer. The presence of the tumor marker alpha-fetoprotein (AFP) in the blood is almost certain to lead to a diagnosis of hepatoma; yet only 60% of people with this liver cancer test positive. Biopsy, most often using a large bore (Trucut) needle, is necessary to confirm the diagnosis.

## Determining Stage

Following a detailed history taking and complete physical examination, blood tests including liver and kidney function and blood coagulation (clotting) studies are administered. Ascites (fluid in the abdomen) is examined for cancer cells. Imaging studies include chest x-ray and abdominal ultrasonography, CT, or MRI. In metastatic cancer to the liver, additional blood and x-ray studies are necessary to determine the site of origin.

## Considerations

If there is a single small cancer, surgery can be curative. Radiation and chemotherapy are of little value. Total hepatectomy and liver transplant are rarely beneficial, and the difficulty in procuring organs for transplant severely curtails its use. The most useful approach is prevention by immunization against hepatitis B and treatment of active cases of hepatitis C with antiviral drugs.

*See also* Bile; Liver Fluke.

# LUNG CANCER

## Overview

The lungs are two sponge-like organs in the chest, in which blood is aerated (oxygen is absorbed and carbon dioxide removed). The right and left lungs are separated by the mediastinum, the center of the chest in front of the spine. The right lung has three natural lobes (divisions), and the left has two. Each lung is connected to the heart by a single, large pulmonary artery and two large pulmonary veins; and both are attached to the windpipe (trachea) by a single large, air passage, the mainstem bronchus. The carina is where the trachea divides into left and right mainstem bronchi. Bronchogenic carcinoma (cancer arising in the lung) is the most common cause of cancer death among men and women in the United States. It occurs in approximately 169,500 adults each year, leading to about 157,400 deaths, and it affects slightly more men than women. Lung cancer is a very lethal cancer.

## Type of Tumor and Spread

Primary lung cancer arises in the lung tissue, most often a bronchus (air passage); this excludes cancer spread to the lung from other sites such as the breast and large bowel. It is categorized as either small cell lung cancer (SCLC) or non-small cell cancer (NSCLC). SCLC is a rapidly growing malignancy that spreads quickly to other organs, especially the brain. NSCLC, the more common variety, is subclassified as squamous cell, adenocarcinoma, and large cell undifferentiated. It doesn't spread as quickly as SCLC, but still spreads faster than most cancers. Advanced cancer can involve the ribs and chest muscles; and when it is located at the top, or apical portion, of the lung (superior sulcus or Pancoast tumor), it can involve nerves to the arm, shoulder, and eye, causing Pancoast syndrome (shoulder and arm pain together with Horner's syndrome).

## Risk Factors

Cigarette smoking is the leading cause of bronchogenic carcinoma, and the risk of cancer increases with the number of cigarettes consumed and years smoked. Although those who stop smoking reduce their chance of developing lung cancer, the risk remains higher than for nonsmokers for as long as 25 years. Nonsmokers exposed to "second-hand smoke" are at increased risk. High levels of radon put uranium miners at an increased risk, and low levels of this radioactive gas in homes may jeopardize occupants, especially if they are smokers. Among asbestos workers, particularly those who smoke, lung cancer and mesothelioma (cancer of the lining of the lung) are the malignancies most often associated with exposure to asbestos.

### Symptoms

Early-stage cancer causes few symptoms, and later problems depend on the size and location of tumor, as well as the presence or absence of spread. Persistent cough is the most common complaint, followed by coughing blood and wheezing. Shortness of breath occurs later, and chest pain is present only after the tumor progresses. Enlarged lymph nodes in the neck above the collarbone indicate locally advanced cancer. Metastasis (spread) to the brain, a common problem with SCLC, causes various problems including headache, nausea, seizures, and weakness. Bone pain results from metastasis involving the skeleton. Other problems, apparently having nothing to do with tumor spread (paraneoplastic syndromes), include pulmonary osteoarthropathy (painless swelling of the finger tips), generalized muscular weakness, and various skin problems including acanthosis nigricans (darkening and thickening of skin in areas that bend or flex, such as the groin, neck, elbows, underarms).

### Diagnosis

A solitary spot or shadow on chest x-ray is often the first indication of primary lung cancer. X-ray evidence of either fluid in the chest or pneumonia indicate more advanced disease. The diagnosis can be made from malignant cells found in the sputum (material coughed up) or fluid drained from the chest as well as from biopsy of lymph nodes in the neck. In most cases, bronchoscopy with biopsy is needed to diagnose cancer. Tumor in the periphery of the lung, beyond the reach of the bronchoscope, is biopsied with a fine needle (FNA) through the chest wall.

### Determining Stage

A thorough history taking and physical examination precede laboratory and other studies. Blood examinations to assess the condition of the patient include a CBC and tests for kidney and liver function. In addition to chest x-rays, chest and abdominal CT are usually done. CT of the brain may also be advised. PET scans are very useful for detecting spread to lymph nodes. Bronchoscopy and in some cases mediastinoscopy are also useful in determining the extent (stage) of disease.

### Considerations

Few individuals today are cured of lung cancer, and new treatment methods are being devised to improve the results. Although NSCLC is curable by surgery when detected and treated at an early stage, this is not common. SCLC is treated with chemotherapy and sometimes with radiation therapy, with about a 10% cure rate if it is found early. NSCLC can be treated with radiation, which is sometimes curative. It responds poorly to chemotherapy. The most obvious way to cure lung cancer is to prevent it by educating the public to the dangers of cigarette smoking. All people, especially teenagers, need to know that cigarette smoking is addictive and that lung cancer rarely occurs in nonsmokers.

*See also* Asbestos; Bronchoalveolar Cancer; Bronchoscopy; Cushing's Syndrome; HER2/*neu*; Mesothelioma (pages 184–185).

## MELANOMA

### Overview

This potentially very serious cancer most often involves the skin, but it also occurs in the eye (ocular melanoma), anus, and vagina. The tumor occurs most often on the leg below the knee in women and on the upper back in men; it rarely affects children. It is becoming more common and affects about 51,400 Americans each year, resulting in approximately 7,800 deaths. Cutaneous melanoma (melanoma of the skin) affects whites about 20 times more often than African Americans, but people with dark skin can also develop the disease.

### Type of Tumor and Spread

Cancer develops in melanocytes, pigment producing cells that give color to the skin, hair, and eyes. Although melanoma expands both horizontally and vertically, downward growth into deeper skin layers and into the fatty subcutaneous tissue leads to involvement of lymph channels and spread to the lymph nodes. The number of adjacent (regional) lymph nodes involved appears directly related to both tumor thickness and tumor ulceration (nonhealing area). Lymph node involvement is followed by metastasis (spread) through the blood to virtually any organ, most often to the brain, lung, or liver. Melanoma is classified into four types:

*Superficial spreading:* The most common variety, which originates in a pre-existing nevus (mole) on sun-exposed areas.

*Nodular:* The second most common variety, which does not arise in a pre-existing skin lesion but appears new.

*Lentigo maligna:* An uncommon melanoma of older people that is characterized by a slow growing, flat, generally large lesion on the face or neck.

*Acral lentiginous:* The most common melanoma of dark-skinned people, which occurs on the palms or sole, or under the nail.

### Risk Factors

Repeated exposure to ultraviolet radiation from the sun, beta rays (UVB) and possibly alpha rays (UVA), appears to promote melanoma in susceptible people.

Individuals especially prone to develop melanoma include fair skinned adults who freckle and sunburn easily, those who live in sunny climates such as the southern United States and Australia, and those who have a family history of melanoma. People with dysplastic nevi (atypical moles) are at increased risk. Severe sunburn around the time of puberty appears to make people, including those without a family history of the melanoma, prone to develop this cancer.

### Symptoms

Any change in a mole that draws attention (changed color, size, or shape; itching, bleeding) is suspicious for superficial spreading melanoma. The appearance of a new, dark colored, skin lesion similar to a blood blister may be the first indication of nodular melanoma. In older people, change in a tan-brown spot on the cheek may indicate lentigo maligna. Any dark spot on the sole, palm, or under the nail not caused by trauma, is possibly acral lentigous melanoma. Unlike blood under the nail from trauma, melanoma in the nail bed (subungual melanoma) does not move with nail growth.

### Diagnosis

Any suspicious lesion that conforms to the "ABCD" of melanoma should be examined and evaluated by a knowledgeable physician.

Asymmetry—cut in two, the halves do not match.

Border irregularity—edges are notched or indented.

Color variation—shades vary from brown, tan, red, blue/black; single or together.

Diameter—usually greater than ¼ inch, the size of a pencil eraser.

Biopsy must include underlying subcutaneous tissue so that the tumor thickness and depth of growth can be determined.

### Determining Stage

Careful history taking and physical examination, with particular attention to the lymph nodes, is followed by blood tests to determine liver function and x-rays of the chest. In advanced-stage melanoma, CT of the chest, abdomen, and/or brain may be needed. Stage depends on careful measurement of tumor thickness and, in some cases, results of lymph node biopsies.

### Considerations

Increased exposure to ultraviolet radiation, possibly from the thinning of the ozone layer, may account for the dramatic increase in cutaneous melanoma over the last 20 years. The use of sunscreens (minimal SPF=15) that block both UVA and UVB rays as well as limiting sun exposure should help to prevent this malignancy. Tanning beds and sun lamps should not be used because they emit ultraviolet radiation, which is hazardous to the skin. Increased awareness of the "ABCDs" of melanoma will enable people to seek treatment at an early stage, when cure is assured with minimal surgery. The American Cancer Society includes examination of the skin in its recommendations for routine cancer-related checkups (*see* Appendix for Cancer Detection Guidelines).

Although cutaneous melanoma is potentially a very serious and sometimes lethal cancer, when discovered at an early stage, it is easily cured by minor surgery. The use of sentinel node biopsy helps define individuals who require regional lymph node removal (lymphadenctomy). Because melanoma appears sensitive to the body's immune (protective) mechanism, immunotherapy may help control the malignancy in both patients who are at increased risk for recurrence after surgery and in those with widespread disease.

*See also* Skin Cancer (pages 199–201); Uveal Melanoma.

## MESOTHELIOMA

### Overview

Mesothelium is the thin layer of cells that covers and protects internal organs. In the chest it forms two layers: visceral pleura covering the lung and parietal pleura lining the chest cavity. The pleural surfaces in contact with each other are lubricated by a thin layer of fluid that allows the lung to expand and contract with each breath. Mesothelium also provides covering for the pericardium (heart) and peritoneum (digestive organs). Cancer arising in mesothelium (mesothelioma) occurs most often in the chest of older white males; and although it is uncommon, it is increasing in occurrence. About 2,000 to 3,000 new cases are diagnosed in the United States each year. It receives a great deal of attention because of its link to asbestos exposure in the workplace.

### Type of Tumor and Spread

Mesothelioma forms either small lumps or flat growths inside the chest, which frequently involve the pericardium, diaphragm, and chest wall (ribs and muscles). Lymph nodes are involved in up to 70% of cases. Spread to other organs includes liver and bone. Death usually occurs from pneumonia or tumor constricting the lung.

### Risk Factors

Although breathing of asbestos particles, particularly in those who smoke cigarettes, is the main cause of pleural mesothelioma, the tumor usually does not appear until 30 to 40 years after first exposure to asbestos.

### Symptoms

Shortness of breath together with vague, mild, chest pain is usually the first indication. As the disease progresses, other symptoms appear, including weight loss, fatigue, fever, and hoarseness.

### Diagnosis

Pleural effusion (fluid between the lung and chest wall) in someone previously exposed to asbestos in the workplace is highly suggestive, but the diagnosis requires pleural biopsy. Endoscopy with a thoracoscope to view the interior of the chest is used to obtain tissue samples. In some cases, opening the chest (thoracotomy) may be needed for diagnosis.

### Determining Stage

Following a detailed history taking and physical examination, blood tests include a CBC and liver function studies. In addition to chest x-rays, CT of the chest is necessary.

### Considerations

It has been difficult for doctors to systematically compare the value of different treatments since mesothelioma is such a rare cancer. Because the outlook for cure is poor, research is focused on developing better methods of drug and radiation therapy. Protecting workers from asbestos should reduce the incidence of this malignancy, although the results will not be seen for many years. Continued surveillance of people exposed to asbestos is essential so that mesothelioma can be discovered early enough to permit successful treatment using current therapy.

*See also* Asbestos; Lung Cancer (pages 180–182).

## MYELOMA

### Overview

Also called multiple myeloma, it is a cancer that begins in the bone marrow. It causes the growth and accumulation of malignant plasma cells (ones derived from B cell lymphocytes—a type of white blood cell or leukocyte), which are active in forming antibodies. Myeloma becomes more common with increased age, most often around age 60. Approximately 14,400 Americans are affected each year, and approximately 11,200 die from the disease.

### Type of Tumor and Spread

Normal plasma cells function as a part of the immune system by producing various antibodies—immunoglobulins or blood proteins that protect against infection. In myeloma, the cells produce only one type of immunoglobulin, called a monoclonal immunoglobulin. The high concentrations of immunoglobulin that often occur in myeloma can lead to kidney failure. Myeloma is also noted for its ability to cause bone damage, with fractures being quite common. Because the body can no longer make normal immunoglobulins, infections are quite common. Anemia, due to bone marrow crowding by myeloma cells, is also common.

### Risk Factors

Most cases of myeloma are not associated with any apparent risk factors. Some studies have found that exposures to petroleum products, dioxin, and atomic radiation appear to increase the occurrence of this disease.

### Symptoms

Bone pain, particularly in the lower back, often occurs first, and fractures may occur as disease progresses. Weakness and paleness due to anemia, or infection may be noticed.

### Diagnosis

Blood tests that indicate anemia and hypercalcemia (increased blood calcium), combined with x-rays showing "punched out" spots in the skeleton are very suggestive. However, the diagnosis of myeloma is usually based upon abnormal proteins (M component) in special blood studies (serum protein electrophoresis) and increased numbers of plasma cells in a bone marrow biopsy. Following a careful history taking and complete physical examination, blood studies include CBC, liver function, and kidney function. Imaging studies include chest x-rays and bone scan.

### Determining Stage

Following a detailed history taking and physical examination, blood tests include testing for levels of albumin, calcium, abnormal monoclonal immunoglobin, hemoglobin, and beta-2-microglobulin. X-rays are used to determine the severity of bone damage.

### Considerations

Myeloma is often responsive to simple chemotherapy; however, no treatment is curative. High-dose chemotherapy with stem cell transplant is an option for younger, healthier patients and may prolong survival. Thalidomide has also proved to be effective for treating myeloma. Other new treatment methods are being investigated to improve the outcome of patients with this cancer.

# NEUROBLASTOMA

## Overview

This very malignant childhood cancer arises in primitive nerve cells that form part of the adrenal gland or in sympathetic nerves adjacent to the spine in either the abdomen or chest. Sympathetic nerves control body functions over which there is no conscious control: heart rate, blood pressure, sweating, pupil size, etc. Although uncommon (about 550 new cases diagnosed each year), it is the most frequent abdominal malignancy in children. The average age at which it occurs is 2 years, and almost 90% of cases are diagnosed by age 6. It affects slightly more boys than girls, and is slightly more common among African-American children than white children. Infants under 1 year old are more likely to be cured than are older children. Neuroblastoma tends to metastasize (spread) widely throughout the body.

## Type of Tumor and Spread

The malignancy is thought to develop from the embryonic (developing) nervous system during the first 2 to 8 weeks of life. About one-third of neuroblastomas start in the adrenal glands, another third begin in the sympathetic nervous system ganglia of the abdomen, and most of the remaining begin in sympathetic ganglia of the chest or neck. Metastasis occurs early and is widespread, especially to the bone, bone marrow, liver, and skin. Most tumors produce the hormones epinephrine and norepinephrine, which are used as tumor markers.

## Risk Factors

Exposure to carcinogenic substances during pregnancy has been suspected by some researchers to increase the risk of neuroblastoma, but none of these have proven to be the cause. This cancer has been found to run in some families, but the majority of patients have no evidence of an inherited predisposition.

## Symptoms

The most common finding is a large, somewhat tender mass extending across the abdomen, which is usually found when the child is bathed. Other indications are decreased appetite, weight loss, vague abdominal pain, fever, not feeling well, and diarrhea. After the tumor has spread, bone pain, skin lumps, and bruising around the eyes may occur.

## Diagnosis

In an infant or a young child a painless lump in the lower part of the abdomen or side is very suggestive. The diagnosis is confirmed by identifying adrenaline-like hormones in blood and urine, together with findings on abdominal CT, ultrasonography, and MRI.

### Determining Stage

Following complete blood count (CBC), urinalysis, liver and kidney function tests, imaging studies include x-rays of chest and skeleton, and bone scan. Bone marrow biopsy is necessary in every case. Evaluation includes genetic and biologic traits (biologic markers) exhibited by the cancer that show it to be favorable or unfavorable (how rapidly it will grow and spread).

### Considerations

Although small infants with early-stage disease may be cured, most children (about 70%) have advanced-stage disease when diagnosed and are less likely to survive. Because widespread neuroblastoma seldom responds to present-day chemotherapy, newer techniques such as stem cell transplant following high-dose chemotherapy, and immunotherapy, are needed to improve the results of today's treatment.

*See also* Childhood Cancer.

## NON-HODGKIN'S LYMPHOMA

### Overview

Non-Hodgkin's lymphoma, usually referred to simply as lymphoma, is a cancer of the lymph nodes and lymphatic tissue. It is seven to eight times more common than Hodgkin's disease, the next most common lymphatic cancer. Although some types of non-Hodgkin's lymphoma are among the most common childhood cancers, over 95% of non-Hodgkin's lymphoma cases occur in adults. The average age at diagnosis is in the early 40s.

In the last 25 years, there has been a greater than 50% increase in the number of cases in the United States; and although this may be due, in part, to the association of lymphoma with AIDS and to better diagnostic techniques, there has been a real overall increase in the incidence of the disease. Unlike Hodgkin's disease, which has become more curable with new treatment methods over the last two decades, some forms of lymphoma have shown little improvement in being permanently controlled. It is estimated that almost 56,200 Americans develop non-Hodgkin's lymphoma each year and about 26,300 die from the disease.

### Type of Tumor and Spread

Non-Hodgkin's lymphoma is a disease of the immune system, usually involving B lymphocytes and, much less often, T lymphocytes. Most cases begin in lymph nodes, but some (extranodal lymphomas) can start in organs other than lymph nodes, such as in the skin, stomach, intestines, lungs, brain, and other organs.

Lymphoma is classified into a number of varieties, which help predict its course and indicate probable response to treatment. The classification system is confusing because there are so many types of the disease and several different systems of classification. The *Working Formulation* method of classifying lymphoma categorizes disease as low grade, intermediate grade, or high grade, based upon expected survival of patients. A newer method of classification, called the *REAL* system, categorizes the types into four classes according to clinical behavior and prognosis *after* treatment and is now considered to be more accurate.

## Risk Factors

Most patients with this disease do not have any known risk factors. Defects in the immune system seen in patients with AIDS and with suppressed immune systems following organ transplant are highly susceptible to developing lymphoma. Viral infection is suspected, particularly in African Burkitt's lymphoma and some forms of T cell lymphoma.

## Symptoms

They vary greatly and are often confused with nonmalignant conditions, particularly infectious mononucleosis. Painless swelling of the lymph nodes, which at first may wax and wane, is the most common symptom. Abdominal complaints include stomach pain, vomiting, and/or passing blood. Skin problems that mimic skin disease (eczema) may be the first indication in some cases (mycosis fungoides). Weight loss, fever, and malaise (feeling poorly) occur as the disease progresses.

## Diagnosis

Although excisional biopsy (lymph node biopsy that removes the entire node) usually is necessary to identify lymphoma, needle biopsy of bone marrow and lymph nodes may reveal lymphoma cells. Biopsy of the stomach and duodenum (using gastroscopy) is used to diagnose lymphoma of these organs. Newer laboratory methods, including flow cytometry and molecular genetic testing, further classify lymphomas into many subtypes, which help predict their behavior and indicate more precise treatment.

## Determining Stage

A careful history taking and physical examination are followed by laboratory studies that include CBC as well as liver and kidney function tests. Imaging studies include chest x-ray, and CT of chest, abdomen, and pelvic area. Bone marrow biopsy is necessary in most cases.

## Considerations

Research continues to develop newer chemotherapy to improve results and cause less adverse effects, especially to the bone marrow. Immunotherapy with the monoclonal antibody rituximab (Rituxan®) is used for low-grade B cell lymphomas that recur or persist after usual therapy. Bone marrow transplant and the use of cytokines to stimulate bone marrow enable high-dose chemotherapy to be used for intermediate- and high-grade lymphomas.

*See also* Burkitt's Lymphoma.

## OVARIAN CANCER

### Overview

The ovaries are a pair of small organs in the female pelvic area. They are the main source of estrogen, and in the nonpregnant state, progesterone. These hormones are responsible for female characteristics including breast and uterine development and regulation of the menstrual cycle. During a woman's reproductive life, between menarche (onset of regular menstrual periods) and menopause (cessation of regular menstruation), the ovaries usually produce a single ovum (egg) approximately every 28 days. Cancer of the ovary is a serious malignancy that most often affects women after menopause, although it may occur earlier. Today, it is the fifth leading cause of cancer deaths in American women. It is estimated that about 23,400 American women are diagnosed with the malignancy each year and almost 14,000 die of it.

### Type of Tumor and Spread

Ninety percent are epithelial ovarian cancer, a variety of adenocarcinoma (gland-forming cancer) that tends to shed cancer cells throughout the pelvis and abdomen. Metastasis (spread) can involve the lymph nodes, but tends to spread to organs such as the liver, lung, and brain late in the course of the disease. However, it often spreads to the surface of the liver and lung. A cancer that resembles ovarian cancer, called primary peritoneal carcinomatosis, can begin in the abdominal cavity even in women who have had their ovaries removed by surgery.

### Risk Factors

Most women with ovarian cancer do not have any known risk factors. However, women with a family history of ovarian cancer are at greater risk for developing ovarian cancer. Also, women with breast cancer are twice as likely to subsequently develop cancer of the ovary. Recently, an inherited mutation (change) in either of two genes (BRCA1 and BRCA2) has been identified in some women with a family history of ovarian and/or breast cancers.

### Symptoms

Unfortunately, there are few symptoms in early-stage disease. Mild abdominal discomfort or pressure, and other digestive disturbances are often so vague as to be ignored. Symptoms of advanced disease include abdominal swelling, and pelvic and abdominal pain. Large tumors cause frequent urination from pressure on the bladder and constipation from pressure on the rectum.

### Diagnosis

Any lower abdominal or pelvic mass felt on pelvic and rectal examination, or ascites (fluid within the abdomen), is highly suspicious. Transvaginal ultrasonography is useful in detecting cancer of the ovary before symptoms arise, and cancer cells found in fluid from the abdomen provide the diagnosis in some cases. Because biopsy of the ovary can spread cancer cells through the abdomen, complete removal of the ovary is used to diagnose cancer confined to the ovary.

### Determining Stage

Following a detailed history taking and complete physical examination, with particular emphasis on pelvic and rectal findings, laboratory studies may include CBC, liver function studies, and the tumor marker CA 125. Among the useful imaging studies are chest x-ray and ultrasonography of the pelvic area.

### Considerations

Surgery is necessary to cure the disease. Because early-stage ovarian cancer is difficult to detect, 75% of women with ovarian cancer have stage II or more advanced disease when first diagnosed. Although recent advances in chemotherapy have greatly increased the life span of women with ovarian cancer, persistent or recurrent disease remains difficult to control. Improved methods are needed to identify cancer limited to the ovary that is likely to be cured. The American Cancer Society includes examination of the ovaries in its recommendations for routine cancer-related checkups (*see* Appendix for Cancer Detection Guidelines). Women at high risk for ovarian cancer (BRCA gene mutation) should consider prophylactic oophorectomy (removal of ovaries) to prevent the malignancy.

*See also* BRCA; CA 125; HER2/*neu*; Oophorectomy.

## PANCREATIC CANCER

### Overview

The pancreas, which lies in front of the spine behind the retroperitoneum (abdominal cavity), is an organ concerned with digestion. It consists of three parts: 1) the larger portion or head, located to the right of the spine, through which the common bile duct that drains bile from the liver to the intestines passes; 2) the mid-portion, or body, in front of the spine; 3) the tail of the organ that lies against the spleen in the left upper part of the abdomen. The pancreas functions as two distinct organs. The major portion or exocrine pancreas produces digestive juice that drains through the pancreatic duct into the duodenum (upper small intestine), where it aids in digesting protein and fats. The endocrine portion of the pancreas is made up of clusters of hormone-producing cells (islet cells) scattered throughout the organ, which produce insulin and glucagon, hormones that affect blood glucose (sugar) levels.

Cancer of the exocrine pancreas accounts for 95% of all pancreatic tumors, and 8 out of 10 occur in people over 60 years old. It is estimated that about 29,200 Americans develop pancreatic cancer each year and approximately 28,900 die of it.

### Type of Tumor and Spread

The most common type (95%) is adenocarcinoma that arises in the ducts in the pancreas. A tumor encroaching on the common bile duct causes jaundice (yellowing of the skin and eyes) by obstructing bile flow from the liver. Metastasis (spread) to adjacent lymph nodes occurs early, usually before symptoms occur. Metastasis to the lung, bone, and brain occurs later.

### Risk Factors

Although scientists still do not know exactly what causes most cases of pancreatic cancer, they have identified several risk factors that can make a person more likely to develop this disease. There are several inherited gene abnormalities known to increase a person's risk of developing pancreatic cancer. Recent studies have found that men and women with BRCA2 mutations have a risk of developing cancer of the pancreas that is 10 to 20 times higher than the risk for the general population. People with p16 mutations may also have a slightly increased risk of developing cancer of the pancreas. A family history of chronic pancreatitis (inflammation of the pancreas) may also be a risk factor. Cigarette smoking also greatly increases the risk. Those who smoke more than two packs a day double their chances of developing this malignancy. A diet high in meats and fat also increases pancreatic cancer risk.

### Symptoms

Pancreatic cancer is termed a "silent cancer" because it causes few symptoms until very advanced. The gradual onset of pain in the upper part of the abdomen, loss of appetite, and weight loss may be noted; but jaundice is usually the first complaint.

### Diagnosis

In an older adult, jaundice together with a mass or swelling in the upper part of the abdomen is most likely due to cancer involving the head of the pancreas, although bile duct and ampullary cancers may cause similar problems. The sudden onset of diabetes sometimes indicates pancreatic malignancy as does painful swelling of the leg due to blood clots.

### Determining Stage

After a complete history taking and physical examination, laboratory studies include liver function and blood clotting studies. Imaging studies include chest x-ray and CT, CT of the abdomen, and possibly a bone scan. Laparoscopy is used to diagnose spread throughout the abdomen.

### Considerations

Surgical therapy for a tumor in the head of the pancreas is a formidable undertaking and is likely to cause postoperative complications, including diabetes and digestive problems. These complications can be minimized when the operation is done by a surgeon who is highly experienced in this procedure, working in a large hospital or cancer center where the procedure is frequently done.

Although surgery is the only means of curing this malignancy, it is most often palliative. Radiation and chemotherapy are also palliative. Because the prognosis for pancreatic cancer is poor, new methods of treatment are needed to improve the results.

*See also* BRCA; Glucagonoma. ,

## PENILE CANCER

### Overview

The penis is the male sex organ that contains the urethra, the small passage through which urine is passed and sperm is ejaculated. Erectile tissue becomes engorged with blood during sexual arousal, causing the organ to become erect for copulation. Cancer of the male sex organ is rare in the United States (1,200 new cases each year); but in other countries, notably Mexico, Paraguay, Uganda, and Southeast Asia, it is a frequent cause of deaths from cancer. Although a malignant tumor of the penis can occur in young men, most are found in males more than 50 years old.

### Type of Tumor and Spread

Penile cancer is usually squamous cell carcinoma that may be preceded by leukoplakia or erythroplakia, a soft white or red spot on the penile skin that cannot be wiped off. Metastasis (spread) occurs early to the lymph node(s) in both groins, and later to nodes in the pelvic area. Metastasis to distant organs, especially the lung and liver, occurs late, often long after the original cancer is treated.

### Risk Factors

Cigarette smoking and having unprotected sex with multiple partners (increasing the likelihood of human papillomavirus infection) are the most important risk factors. Some have suggested that circumcision offers some protection from developing the disease by contributing to improved hygiene, but this has not been proven.

### Symptoms

A painless wart-like growth or sore on the tip of the penis is the most common. But in some men, enlarged lymph node(s) in the groin (inguinal area) may be the first complaint.

### Diagnosis

Any growth or sore on the penis of an older uncircumcised male is very suspicious; especially if there is an enlarged lymph node in the groin. Biopsy of the tumor furnishes both the diagnosis and depth of tumor penetration (invasion), and needle biopsy reveals spread to lymph nodes in the groin.

### Determining Stage

Following a history taking and careful physical examination, laboratory studies include liver function tests. Imaging studies include chest x-ray and pelvic CT.

### Considerations

In recent years, much progress has been made in treating penile cancer, and surgery is the most common treatment for all stages. At this time, controversy exists over the need for removing lymph nodes in all cases. In the future, sentinel node biopsy may indicate only nodes containing cancer that need to be removed.

*See also* Human Papillomavirus.

## PROSTATE CANCER

### Overview

The prostate is a walnut-size gland at the base of the bladder. It is a part of the male reproductive system that produces semen, the thick fluid in which sperm are ejaculated. Today, prostate cancer is the most frequently diagnosed malignant tumor in American men, and only lung cancer causes more deaths in this group. It appears to be more common than in the past, especially among African Americans (70% more often than in white men), and it is estimated that more than 198,000 men (approximately 10% of the males in the United States) develop the disease each year. Because prostate cancer is a malignancy of older men (more than 70% of all prostate cancers are diagnosed in men over the age of 65) and often is very slow growing, it can be said that more men die with prostate cancer than because of it. Although it is estimated that this disease kills about 31,500 American men each year, 93% of all men diagnosed with prostate cancer survive at least 5 years, and 72% survive at least 10 years. African-American men are twice as likely as white men to die from the disease.

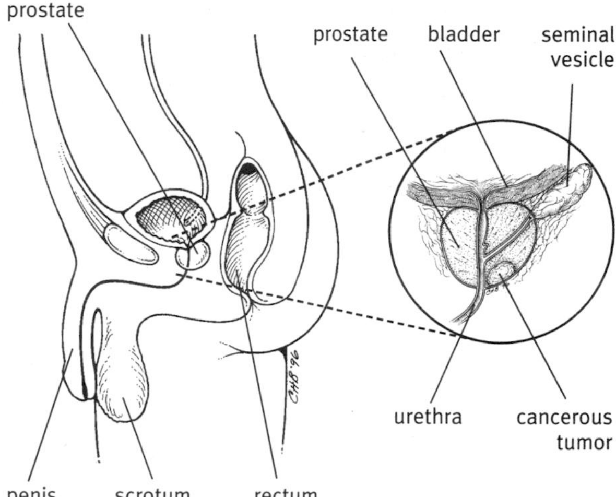


### Type of Tumor and Spread

The tumor is almost always adenocarcinoma. Initial spread beyond the prostate is to surrounding tissue in the pelvic area and nearby lymph nodes. Metastasis via the blood usually occurs first to the bone.

### Risk Factors

Genetic changes (DNA mutations) inherited from a parent appear to be responsible for about 5% to 10% of prostate cancers. Men who eat a lot of fat in their diet also have a greater chance of developing prostate cancer. Regular physical activity and maintaining a healthy weight may help reduce prostate cancer risk.

### Symptoms

There are usually no apparent symptoms in the early stages of the disease. Most severe problems are related to bone metastasis and include back pain and stiffness, and occasionally, fractures. Tumor growth within the gland itself may block urine flow from the bladder, which leads to difficulty starting urination, frequent urination (especially at night), a less forceful urinary stream, painful urination, and hematuria (blood in the urine). These urinary symptoms are identical to those caused by noncancerous enlargement of the prostate gland or benign prostatic hypertrophy (BPH). A urologist, who specializes in treating urinary problems, must determine if the problems are cancer-related. Impotence may also be another indication.

### Diagnosis

A lump or mass in the prostate found on a rectal examination has been the usual means of detecting the disease. Today, however, increased levels in blood of the tumor marker, prostate-specific antigen (PSA), are often the first indication of prostate malignancy. A metastasis in the lower spine or pelvic bones in an older man is very suspicious. In all cases, the correct diagnosis requires biopsy of the prostate through the rectum with a large bore (Trucut) needle, which causes little discomfort and few complications.

### Determining Stage

Following a detailed history taking and careful physical examination, blood studies include PSA as well as kidney and liver function. Imaging studies include chest x-ray, CT or MRI of the pelvic area, and bone scan. Precise staging depends on biopsy of the pelvic lymph nodes at surgery.

### Considerations

Following screening guidelines can improve the chances of survival (*see* Appendix for Cancer Detection Guidelines). The use of PSA to detect very early cancer has increased the number of men successfully treated for the malignancy and has improved the outlook for those with the disease. Whether every man with elevated PSA needs therapy is debatable. The ideal way to treat all stages of prostate cancer is far from settled. New and different methods of prostate surgery and radiation therapy are needed to lessen the complications of altered sexual, bladder, and rectal function that often accompany present-day therapy. In elderly men, early-stage prostate cancer may not need treatment unless the disease progresses.

*See also* Prostatectomy; Prostate-Specific Antigen.

## RETINOBLASTOMA

### Overview

The retina is the innermost layer of the eye, which converts light into nerve impulses sent to the brain through the optic nerve. Retinoblastoma is a relatively uncommon cancer of younger children that affects about 200 children each year, 80% of whom are diagnosed before age 4. Although the tumor usually affects only one eye, it can involve both in one-fourth of the cases. Because retinoblastoma has not typically spread outside the eyeball when first treated, over 90% of children with this malignancy survive for more than 5 years. In some cases, the tumor has been known to undergo spontaneous regression (completely disappear without treatment).

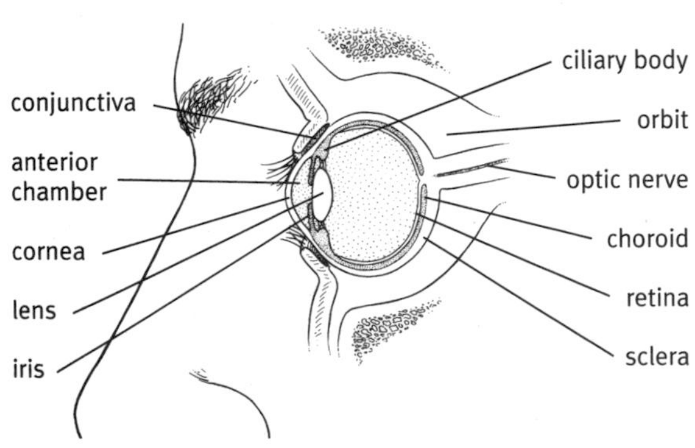


### Type of Tumor and Spread

The tumor is made up of cells that somewhat resemble retinal cells present in the eye of the embryo soon after conception. Tumor growth involves other layers of the eye, and later, of the surrounding tissues. Multiple tumors are often present within the eye. Extensive growth may involve the meninges (covering of the brain) and cause metastasis (spread) of malignant cells in the spinal fluid. Metastasis through blood to distant sites includes the lung, bone, and bone marrow.

**Risk Factors**

Chromosome changes due to an abnormal "retinoblastoma gene" have been identified. About 40% of the cases are hereditary and can affect one or both eyes, while nonhereditary retinoblastomas nearly always affect only one eye. The cause of the nongenetic (sporadic) form of this cancer is unknown.

**Symptoms**

A white spot in the center of the pupil (leukocoria or cat eye reflex) is most often the first problem noticed, but a crossed, or reddened eye, and impaired vision may be the initial problem.

**Diagnosis**

Retinoblastoma is typically identified through careful eye examination under anesthesia, which reveals the chalky white tumor. Because eye infection due to the parasite *Toxocara canis* may be confused with retinoblastoma, the test for the parasite may be needed to determine the cause of leukocoria.

**Determining Stage**

Following a careful physical examination, blood studies include CBC and liver and kidney function tests. Imaging studies of the eye and surrounding tissue, with ultrasonography, CT or MRI, determine the extent of disease, as does examination of spinal fluid. Bone scan may be needed in advanced cases.

**Considerations**

Because retinoblastoma is rare, few doctors except those in specialty eye hospitals and major children's cancer centers have much experience in treating these patients. Surgery, radiation, and chemotherapy are all used in therapy, and laser and cryotherapy may be used in early stage disease. Because only 10% of children with extraocular tumor (spread outside the eye) survive without cancer for 5 years, new methods of multidrug chemotherapy are being investigated to improve these poor treatment results. All children with retinoblastoma, especially the hereditary form, are at increased risk of developing second malignancies, particularly bone tumors within irradiated tissue; and they need to be followed, even as adults, to detect and treat secondary cancers.

Genetic testing should be done on all patients with retinoblastoma, and parents and siblings of affected children should have regular eye examinations to detect early eye cancer.

*See also* Childhood Cancer; Leukocoria.

# SALIVARY GLAND CANCER

## Overview

The major and minor salivary glands are oral glands that produce fluids that lubricate the mouth, soften and dilute food, and convert starch to sugar. The major glands are composed of three pairs of small organs that produce saliva. The parotids, located in front of each ear, are the largest and are most often the site of cancer. The smaller submandibular glands, located under each side of the lower jaw, have a higher percentage of malignant tumors than the other glands. The sublingual glands, the smallest of the major glands, are in the floor of the mouth in front of the tongue and are least often the site of cancer. The minor salivary glands are tiny glands scattered beneath the mucosa (lining) of the nose, throat, and palate (roof of the mouth), which mainly secrete mucous. Cancer of both major and minor glands comprises only 6% to 7% of all head and neck malignant tumors.

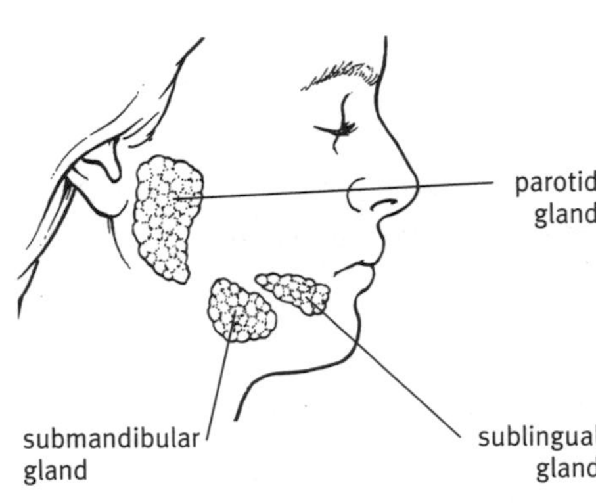


## Type of Tumor and Spread

These uncommon cancers are a dissimilar group of at least eight different types, which vary from very slow to very fast growing tumors. Salivary gland tumors are given a numeric grade of 1, 2, or 3 based on their appearance under a microscope. High-grade cancers that bear little resemblance to normal salivary gland tissue occur most often in older people and are likely to involve surrounding tissue, skin, nerve, and bone. They quickly spread to lymph nodes and distant organs.

## Risk Factors

Exposure to radioactive substances and radiation treatment to the head and neck increases the risk of salivary gland cancer. Some studies have found that industrial exposure to certain metals (nickel alloy dust) or minerals (silica dust) is associated with increased risk. Tobacco use and high-fat diets may also be risk factors for some types of salivary gland cancer.

## Symptoms

In parotid cancer, painless swelling in front of the ear is often the first, although drooping of one corner of the mouth or numbness of part of the face may be noted. Cancer of the submandibular gland usually causes painless swelling beneath the lower jaw. Cancer of the sublingual gland produces a lump in the floor of the mouth in front of the tongue. Minor salivary gland cancers cause lumps in the mucosa (lining) of the mouth, nose, and throat.

### Diagnosis

Because all salivary gland tumors need to be removed, the diagnosis of cancer is often not made until surgery. When a mass that is highly suspected to be cancerous cannot be removed because of its size or another medical problem, biopsy by fine needle aspiration (FNA) can be used to identify the tumor.

### Determining Stage

A careful physical examination is followed by imaging studies that include a chest x-ray. In addition, CT or MRI of the head and neck are obtained if the tumor appears to involve surrounding tissue.

### Considerations

New methods of therapy combining neutron radiation and chemotherapy before or after surgery are needed to improve the results of advanced and rapidly growing salivary gland cancers. Because present-day therapy of recurrent and widespread disease is rarely successful, new treatment methods including immunotherapy are being studied.

*See also* Head and Neck Cancer (pages 170–172).

## SKIN CANCER (Nonmelanoma)

### Overview

The skin is made up of two layers: epidermis (outer layer) and dermis (inner layer). Either of these layers can give rise to cancer, although the great majority begin in the epidermis. Skin cancer (including melanoma and nonmelanoma) is the most common human malignancy, which most often affects light-skinned, older people, usually on areas exposed to sunlight, especially the face, ears, back of hands, and scalp. However, the genitals and other parts of the body may be affected. Men are more likely than women to develop skin cancer. Although no statistics are kept on nonmelanoma skin cancer, it is estimated that more than 1.3 million new cases occur annually in the United States. Even though death is rarely caused by skin cancer other than melanoma (about 2,000 deaths each year), serious problems can result from recurrent cancer, which occurs in 10% of patients.

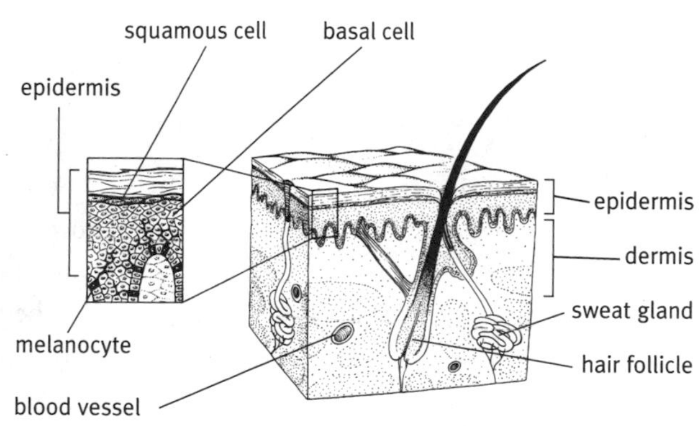

## Type of Tumor and Spread

The majority are classified as either basal cell or squamous cell carcinoma. Basal cell, the most prevalent human cancer, is a slow growing tumor; and although it is capable of causing extensive destruction and even death, it rarely spreads to lymph nodes or other organs. Squamous cell cancer can be either fast or slow growing, and it is likely to metastasize after penetrating deeper into the dermis and fatty subcutaneous tissue beneath the skin. Spread is first to adjacent lymph nodes.

## Risk Factors

The accumulated lifetime dose of solar radiation (ultraviolet radiation from the sun) appears responsible. Fair-skinned people who work outdoors and tend to burn, rather than tan, and who develop precancerous age spots (solar or actinic keratosis) are particularly at risk. The risk of skin cancer is more than 20 times higher for whites than for African Americans. People who have had radiation therapy have a higher risk of developing nonmelanoma skin cancer in the area that received treatment. Also, individuals with chronic skin irritation from long-standing leg ulcers caused by varicose veins, burn scars, and osteomyelitis (bone infection) are at increased risk of squamous cell cancer. Xeroderma pigmentosum, a skin condition appearing in childhood, which causes extreme sensitivity to sunlight, leads to skin cancer in all cases. Exposure to arsenic, a heavy metal used in making some insecticides, in pressure-treated wood products, and naturally found in drinking water in some parts of the world, increases the risk of developing nonmelanoma skin cancer. People with an altered immune system, including those given drugs to prevent organ rejection, and those with AIDS, are more at risk for developing skin cancer.

## Symptoms

Squamous cell carcinoma appears most often as a nonhealing sore or ulcer that rapidly increases in size. Enlarged lymph node(s) due to spread of cancer may be first noticed. Basal cell cancer usually begins as a small, pink or skin-colored pimple that slowly enlarges to form an ulcer with rolled up edges and a depressed center.

## Diagnosis

Because skin cancers appear in many different forms, it can be difficult to accurately identify; however, any skin lesion that undergoes a change in size, shape, or color is suspicious. Any sore that does not heal and continues to bleed may indicate more advanced cancer. Biopsy is necessary for diagnosis; and for small cancers, excisional biopsy that removes the entire lesion is usually all that is needed.

### Determining Stage

Physical examination, with particular attention to the lymph nodes, is followed by laboratory studies that include liver function studies in cases of advanced cancer. Chest x-ray is advised in advanced disease, and CT of the area of the tumor may be indicated in head and neck lesions.

### Considerations

Fortunately, most basal cell and squamous cell carcinomas can be completely cured by fairly minor surgery. Using sunscreens, seeking shade, protecting the body with clothing, and avoiding prolonged sun exposure lower the risk of solar radiation injury to the skin and lessen the number of skin cancers. Retinoid cream, similar to vitamin A, can be used to reduce the likelihood of skin cancer developing from a keratosis.

*See also* Kaposi's Sarcoma; Melanoma (pages 182–184).

## SMALL INTESTINE CANCER

### Overview

The small bowel or small intestine is the part of the digestive tract where food is mixed with bile and other enzymes and broken down into simple compounds to be absorbed. It begins at the pylorus (stomach outlet) and ends at the cecum, the first part of the large intestine or colon. Overall, it is approximately 22 feet in length. The first 10 inches (the duodenum) is where bile and pancreatic juice enter through a small opening, the common bile duct. The mid-portion (jejunum), which is about 10 feet long and the terminal portion (ileum), which is only slightly longer, are where digested nutrients are absorbed. Cancer of the small intestine is 30 to 60 times less frequent than cancer of the large bowel, and accounts for only about 1% to 3% of gastrointestinal (GI) malignant tumors. It occurs mainly after age 60; and about 5,300 new cases are diagnosed each year in the United States, leading to approximately 1,100 deaths.

### Type of Tumor and Spread

Adenocarcinoma of the intestinal mucosa (lining) is the most common malignant tumor in the small intestine, with 90% occurring in the duodenum and jejunum. Metastasis (spread) occurs when tumor penetrates or invades the intestinal wall to involve lymphatics and lymph nodes adjacent to blood vessels. In duodenal carcinoma, adjacent nodes include those around the pancreas. People with small bowel cancer are at increased risk for developing second, unrelated malignant tumors.

### Risk Factors

A diet rich in red meat and salt-cured or smoked foods as well as a high-fat diet may be risk factors. People with inflammatory bowel disease and Peutz-Jeghers syndrome are more likely to develop carcinoma of the small bowel.

### Symptoms

Tumors in the small intestine cause few symptoms until they reach a very advanced stage. They vary considerably depending on location and extent of cancer. Jaundice, cramping abdominal pain, weight loss, nausea, and passing or vomiting blood are indications. Persistent abdominal pain or a mass in the abdomen indicate advanced disease.

### Diagnosis

It is not unusual for the diagnosis to take several months, and in some cases may not be made until abdominal surgery. Present-day x-ray studies (upper GI series with small bowel follow-through) are not very revealing, and abdominal CT is not highly accurate in diagnosing small bowel tumors. Endoscopy to visualize and biopsy tumor is limited to the duodenum and lower (terminal) part of the ileum.

### Determining Stage

A thorough history taking and complete physical examination are followed by laboratory tests, including CBC and liver function. Imaging studies include chest x-rays and abdominal CT. Gastroscopy and colonoscopy are commonly advised.

### Considerations

Surgery is the only way to cure the disease. Because present-day endoscopy allows only the duodenum and terminal ileum to be biopsied, newer endoscopic methods are needed to evaluate the entire small intestine.

*See also* Colorectal Cancer (pages 163–165); Peutz-Jeghers Syndrome.

## SOFT TISSUE CANCER

### Overview

Soft tissue is made up of cells (other than bone) that support, connect, and surround organs or body parts and includes muscles, fat, tendons, blood vessels, and nerves. Cancer of soft tissue is not a single disease, but is a variety of malignant tumors that can arise anywhere in the body, especially the arms and legs. Although it is estimated that only 8,700 Americans develop soft tissue sarcoma each year, it remains a serious disease because approximately 4,400 people die of it. Unlike most malignancies, which differ markedly in adults and children, soft tissue cancers are often similar in all age groups, although older people seem to fare less well following treatment. These malignancies account for a large percentage of deaths due to cancer in children less than 15 years old.

### Type of Tumor and Spread

All soft tissue cancers are sarcomas, which are classified according to the site in which they arise and their grade (how much the cancer resembles the tissue from which it arises). The three most common are *malignant fibrous histiocytoma* that involves tissues that support, cushion, and connect body parts; *liposarcoma* that arises in fat; and *leiomyosarcoma* that occurs in the smooth muscle of internal organs and blood vessels. The most common soft tissue sarcomas of infants and children are *rhabdomyosarcoma*, involving voluntary muscle connected to bone, and *peripheral primitive neuroectodermal tumor,* involving nerves outside the brain and spinal cord. Although malignancies of soft tissue seldom spread to lymph nodes, lymphatic spread is more likely to occur in childhood sarcomas. In all age groups, the tendency of soft tissue sarcomas to spread or metastasize depends on size and tumor grade. The poor outlook for soft tissue sarcomas is due mainly to their tendency to invade surrounding tissue early on and spread via blood to the lungs. However, people with small tumors who receive optimum therapy can expect a favorable outcome.

### Risk Factors

A genetic cause has been identified in some instances, particularly in children, and in patients with AIDS, which destroys the body's immune (protective) system and is associated with Kaposi's sarcoma. Previous cancer treatment also has been implicated. Prior radiation therapy is associated with sarcoma in irradiated tissues, especially following treatment of breast and cervical cancers and of lymphoma. In women with severe postoperative arm swelling following mastectomy, radiation to the lymph nodes under the arm has been linked to angiosarcoma of the lymph channels and small blood vessels in the skin of the arm (Stewart-Treves syndrome). In addition, exposure to industrial chemicals (herbicides, wood preservatives, compounds used in plastics manufacture) appears responsible in some cases.

### Symptoms

Because most sarcomas occur in the extremities, a painless, enlarging lump in the arm, leg, or thigh that is often blamed on injury is usually the first indication. Most lumps (two-thirds) are painless. Soft tissue tumor in the abdomen can cause abdominal pain or rectal or urinary bleeding depending on the organ involved. A painless mass or lump in the abdomen may be noted.

### Diagnosis

Any persistent or enlarging lump in an arm, leg, or deep within the abdomen, which is painful, is very suspicious. However, the definitive diagnosis requires a biopsy, obtained either by incisional biopsy (removing a piece of tumor) or using a large bore (Trucut) needle. It is critical that the biopsy be planned so that the resulting scar can be removed with the tumor if additional surgery is needed.

### Determining Stage

An accurate history taking and complete physical examination are followed by blood studies that include CBC and a liver function test. Imaging studies include chest x-ray and CT as well as CT or MRI of the tumor site.

### Considerations

Treatment combining surgery, radiation, and chemotherapy has greatly improved the survival for those with soft tissue sarcomas, but newer methods of radiation therapy and chemotherapy are needed to further improve results. Immunotherapy is being studied to improve survival in widespread or recurrent sarcoma.

*See also* Kaposi's Sarcoma; Leiomyosarcoma; Liposarcoma; Malignant Fibrous Histiocytoma; Neurofibrosarcoma; Rhabdomyosarcoma; Sarcoma.

## STOMACH CANCER

### Overview

The stomach is the muscular, sac-like, digestive organ between the lower end of the esophagus and the first part of the small intestine (duodenum) where swallowed food is mixed with acid and digestive enzymes. Stomach cancer, also known as gastric cancer, is an adult malignancy that more often affects men over age 50. About 21,700 Americans are diagnosed with stomach cancer each year, leading to approximately 12,800 deaths. Once the most common internal malignant tumor in the United States, stomach cancer incidence has decreased dramatically over the past 50 years. Proximal gastric cancer (cancer of the upper portion of the stomach) is increasing in white males, unlike cancer of the remainder of the stomach, which most often affects African Americans and is becoming less common. In Japan, Chile, and Costa Rica, stomach cancer remains the leading cause of deaths due to cancer.

### Type of Tumor and Spread

The most common type (90% to 95%) is adenocarcinoma that forms an ulcer or tumor in the inner mucosa (lining) of the stomach. Two distinct types of carcinoma are recognized: intestinal and diffuse, the latter of which is a faster growing and more aggressive variety. In the past, gastric cancer occurred most often in the lower end of the stomach, but today it is found equally in the upper part adjacent to the esophagus (gastroesophageal or GE junction). Spread can occur through lymph channels to adjacent nodes, via blood to distant organs, through involvement of the esophagus or duodenum, or penetration through the stomach to involve abdominal organs.

### Risk Factors

Carcinogens (cancer-causing substances) in the diet are considered the most likely risk factor. An increased risk of stomach cancer is associated with tobacco and alcohol use as well as diets containing large amounts of smoked foods, salted fish and meat, certain foods high in starch that are also low in fiber, and pickled vegetables. A recently recognized bacterium, *Helicobacter pylori,* which causes chronic stomach irritation or gastritis, is suspected to play a role in some cases. Both pernicious anemia and atrophic gastritis, noncancerous conditions associated with decreased stomach acid, predispose people to stomach cancer. Partial gastrectomy (removal of the lower part of the stomach) for nonmalignant ulcer disease increases the risk, possibly by allowing bile and intestinal juice to flow up into the stomach and irritate the lining. For unknown reasons, blood type A predisposes people to gastric cancer. There is also a hereditary form of stomach cancer.

### Symptoms

Often few problems occur until cancer is in an advanced stage, and then only vague indigestion, loss of appetite, and weight loss may be noted. In some cases, a tired or weak feeling due to anemia from unsuspected bleeding may be the only complaint. An advanced tumor in the proximal (upper) stomach may cause swallowing difficulty, and in the distal (lower) stomach may produce a full feeling and vomiting.

### Diagnosis

Every stomach ulcer is potentially cancerous, and any growth or mass felt in the upper part of the abdomen is suspicious. Enlarged lymph nodes in the lower part of the neck often indicate spread or metastasis. Gastroscopy to view and biopsy the interior of the stomach is often the first diagnostic procedure.

### Determining Stage

A thorough history taking, physical examination, and biopsy are followed by blood studies including CBC and liver function studies. Chest x-ray and CT of the abdomen are necessary. More recently, endoscopic ultrasonography and laporoscopy are used preoperatively to stage the tumor.

### Considerations

Surgery is the only means of curing gastric cancer. In the United States and other countries, the treatment of stomach cancer is not very effective (the overall 5-year survival rate is 21%), except in early-stage disease, which is not often diagnosed. Different treatment methods combining chemotherapy, radiation therapy, and immunotherapy are being evaluated to improve the results of present-day therapy.

*See also* Gastroscope; Gastroscopy.

## TESTICULAR CANCER

### Overview

The testicles (testes) are the primary male sex glands, located in the scrotum or sac beneath the penis. They produce and store sperm, and are the main source of testosterone, the hormone responsible for male sex organ development and masculine characteristics including body shape, muscular development, hair pattern, and voice depth. Testicular cancer most often occurs in young men between the ages of 15 and 40. It usually affects only one side. Over the last 20 years, it has become significantly more common in white males. It affects about 7,200 American men each year, leading to almost 400 deaths. The treatment of cancer of the testicle is very successful, with over 90% of all patients being cured.

### Type of Tumor and Spread

Almost all (over 90%) arise in germ cells (embryonic cells that give rise to cells that produce sperm) and are classified as either seminoma or nonseminoma. The latter includes the subtypes embryonal carcinoma, choriocarcinoma, teratoma, and yolk cell tumor. Testicular cancers tend to metastasize (spread) first to lymph nodes deep within the abdomen and later through blood to the lungs, liver, and bone. When first diagnosed, approximately half of those with nonseminoma have cancer spread outside the scrotum.

### Risk Factors

Approximately 10% of those affected have a history of cryptorchism (failure of one or both testicles to descend into the scrotum, a process that normally takes place before birth). There is apparently no increased risk of cancer developing in an undescended testis if it is brought down surgically into the scrotum before age 6. Testicular cancer is also sometimes associated with a family history of the disease.

### Symptoms

A small, hard, lump or swelling in one testicle is usually the first indication in most cases (90%). A heavy feeling or discomfort in the scrotum may be noted.

### Diagnosis

Ultrasonography is used to determine if the lump is a solid tumor mass in the testes, in which case the entire gland is removed by an operation in the groin (inguinal orchiectomy) to obtain the diagnosis. Biopsy through the scrotum should not be done because of the possibility of spreading cancer cells. Removal of the testis not only furnishes the diagnosis, but also provides primary treatment in many cases.

### Determining Stage

Following a detailed history taking and physical examination, blood tests include liver function studies, and tumor markers alpha-fetoprotein (AFP) and human chorionic gonadotropin (hCG). Imaging studies include a chest x-ray and CT of the chest, abdomen, and pelvis.

### Considerations

Treatment consists of surgery, combined with radiation and chemotherapy according to the type and stage of disease. Therapy of testicular cancer is among the most successful treatments of adult malignancies; and in early-stage disease, over 95% of patients are cured. The American Cancer Society includes testicular examination in its recommendations for routine cancer-related checkups (*see* Appendix for Cancer Detection Guidelines).

*See also* Germ Cell Cancer.

## THYROID CANCER

### Overview

The thyroid is a hormone-producing (endocrine) gland in the front of the neck that produces several hormones that regulate metabolism (chemical and physical processes that control the body's growth and energy). Thyroid growth and activity are in turn regulated by thyroid-stimulating hormone (TSH) from the pituitary, a small gland beneath the brain. Cancer of the thyroid receives attention because it occurs frequently in young adults and occasionally in children and teenagers. About 19,500 Americans develop thyroid cancer each year, leading to 1,300 deaths. It is more than three times more common in women than men. Malignant tumors that appear identical under the microscope may be far more aggressive and difficult to control in older people than in younger individuals.

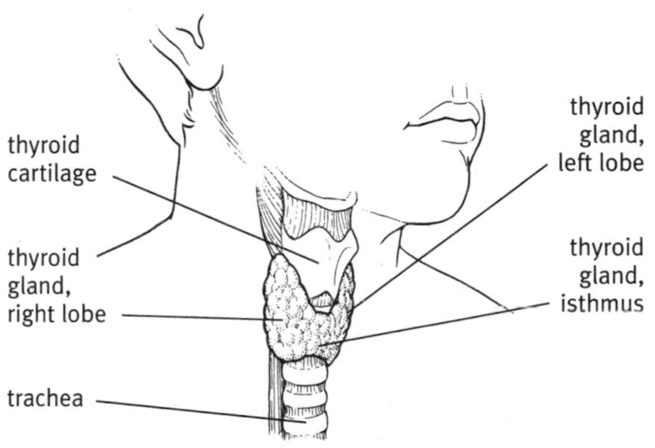

## Type of Tumor and Spread

There are five distinct cancers of the thyroid that have been identified. Those comprised of more than one tumor variety are classed according to the prominent cell type identified under the microscope.

*Papillary carcinoma:* The most common variety, especially in children and young adults, is prone to spread to cervical lymph nodes in the neck and rarely involves lung, bone, and other organs.

*Follicular carcinoma:* The next most common tumor can spread through the blood to the bone and lung and usually does not involve lymph nodes in the neck. Hurthle cell carcinoma, a subtype, is a very uncommon tumor that acts similar to follicular carcinoma.

*Medullary carcinoma:* An endocrine cancer that produces the hormone calcitonin, and may be associated with inherited multiple endocrine neoplasia (MEN) syndrome. Spread occurs to lymph nodes in the neck and later to nodes in the chest. Spread via the blood is to the bone, lung, liver, and adrenal glands.

*Anaplastic (undifferentiated) carcinoma:* An uncommon, rapidly growing malignancy of older people, which involves adjacent neck structures including the trachea and esophagus. Spread is to both lymph nodes and distant organs.

*Thyroid lymphoma:* The thyroid is an uncommon, but possible, location for lymphoma to develop.

## Risk Factors

One proven contributing factor is radiation, either from x-ray therapy to the head and neck during childhood or following exposure to atomic bomb blasts or nuclear accidents. Malignancies resulting from childhood therapy are very curable. Follicular carcinoma and particularly anaplastic carcinoma are associated with goiter (a chronic noncancerous thyroid enlargement often due to lack of iodine in the diet). People with certain inherited medical conditions, such as Gardner's syndrome, are also at higher risk of thyroid cancer. About 20% of medullary thyroid carcinomas result from inheriting an abnormal gene.

## Symptoms

A solitary nodule (single mass or lump) in the front of the neck is the most common symptom. But some people, especially children, may first notice one or more lumps in the side of the neck apart from the thyroid due to cancer that has spread to lymph node(s). Older adults may become aware of a sudden rapid growth in a long-standing goiter. Hoarseness from vocal cord paralysis occurs in cancer involving either of the two nerves to the larynx (recurrent laryngeal nerves) that stimulate the vocal cords. Difficulty swallowing, breathing problems, and a persistent cough may also be indications.

### Diagnosis

Biopsy with a fine needle (fine needle aspiration) is most useful for diagnosing papillary, anaplastic, and medullary carcinoma. However, biopsy using a large bore (Trucut) needle or complete removal of a nodule (lump) is usually necessary to distinguish follicular cancer from the benign tumor known as follicular adenoma. Thyroid scans and ultrasonography often suggest whether a thyroid mass is benign or malignant. Thyroid tumors that take up excess radioisotope (hot nodule) and cysts that take up little or no isotope (cold nodule) are rarely malignant; however, neither imaging study can definitely identify cancer.

### Determining Stage

Careful history taking, especially regarding childhood exposure to radiation, and physical examination are followed by blood studies, which include calcitonin levels when medullary carcinoma is suspected. Imaging studies include chest x-ray and ultrasonography.

### Considerations

The American Cancer Society includes examination of the thyroid in its recommendations for routine cancer-related checkups (*see* Appendix for Cancer Detection Guidelines). Although papillary and follicular carcinomas are among the most curable of all malignancies, anaplastic cancer, which is extremely rare, remains incurable. Surgery is the treatment for all carcinomas except the anaplastic variety, and it may be accompanied by radiation and hormone therapy depending upon the type and stage of disease. Stopping x-ray treatment for benign childhood conditions, including acne and enlarged tonsils, has reduced the number of adults with papillary and follicular cancers. In families with medullary cancer, the presence of increased calcitonin in family members identifies those with C cell hyperplasia, the forerunner of medullary cancer, who require total thyroidectomy to prevent cancer.

*See also* Follicular Carcinoma; Head and Neck Cancer (pages 170–172).

## VAGINAL CANCER

### Overview

The vagina or birth canal is part of the female reproductive system that connects the lower portion of the uterus, or womb, to the vulva or external female genitals. Cancer of the vagina is rare (about 2,100 new cases each year) and accounts for only 3% of malignant tumors of the female sex organs. Most malignancies that involve the birth canal do not originate in the vagina but are usually spread from cancer of the uterus or the cervix. Although primary vaginal cancer occurs most often in women over age 50, a rare variety, clear cell adenocarcinoma, affects women at an average age of 19.

### Type of Tumor and Spread

Eighty-five to ninety percent are squamous cell carcinomas that form an ulcer or a cauliflower-like growth in the vagina. Metastasis (spread) to adjacent organs involves the bladder, rectum, and lymph nodes in the pelvic and groin areas. About 5% to 10% of vaginal cancers are adenocarcinomas. Although squamous cell cancers seldom metastasize outside the pelvic area, clear cell adenocarcinoma in young females tends to spread to distant sites such as the lung and liver. Clear cell carcinoma that affects young girls has been linked to the synthetic female hormone diethylstilbestrol (DES), which was given to their mothers during the first 4 months of pregnancy to prevent miscarriage. DES has not been used in women in the United States since 1971. The more common squamous carcinoma may be related to papillomaviruses that cause genital warts. In some instances vaginal cancer is known to follow prior radiation therapy to the pelvic area. About 2% to 3% of vaginal cancers are sarcomas, which form deep in the wall of the vagina, not on its surface epithelium.

### Symptoms

Vaginal bleeding or discharge, particularly after intercourse, is usual; however, in early-stage disease there may be few symptoms. Pelvic pain, constipation, and painful urination may be caused by advanced cancer.

### Diagnosis

Findings on pelvic examination usually indicate cancer, although it may be difficult to determine whether tumor originates in the vagina or the cervix. Biopsy of the lesion under local anesthesia gives the correct diagnosis.

### Determining Stage

Following history taking and complete physical examination, evaluation of the vagina and cervix is necessary using a colposcope, a lighted magnifying instrument. Blood tests include kidney function studies. Chest x-rays and pelvic CT are usual, and pelvic MRI may be helpful. Cystoscopy to examine the bladder, and sigmoidoscopy to evaluate the rectum may be necessary in advanced cases.

### Considerations

Vaginal cancer is curable in the majority of cases because it usually causes symptoms at an early stage and is easily recognized on a Pap test or pelvic examination. The American Cancer Society includes pelvic examination in its recommendations for routine cancer-related checkups (*see* Appendix for Cancer Detection

Guidelines). Carcinoma in situ of the vagina is more difficult to treat because spread to lymph nodes and other sites is often present when the disease is diagnosed. In the future, treatment combining chemotherapy with low-dose radiation may reduce the problems presently associated with high-dose radiation therapy.

*See also* Clear Cell Vaginal Cancer; Human Papillomavirus.

## VULVAR CANCER

### Overview

The vulva or external female genitalia is comprised of the labia (large and small vaginal lips), clitoris, vaginal opening, and urethra (bladder opening). Cancer of the vulva accounts for only a small fraction of malignant tumors of a woman's reproductive organs (about 4%). About 3,600 cases are diagnosed each year, leading to approximately 800 deaths. When detected early, it is highly curable. It occurs most often in the poorer classes. Three-fourths of women with vulvar cancer are over the age of 50, although carcinoma in situ, the premalignant forerunner of most of vulvar cancer, occurs in women 15 to 20 years younger. Some research suggests that this cancer is becoming more common, particularly in young women, but this has not yet been proven.

### Type of Tumor and Spread

Approximately 90% to 95% of vulvar cancers are squamous cell carcinomas that develop very slowly over many years from carcinoma in situ. The labia, clitoris, and urethra area are most often involved, usually with tumor that forms an enlarging sore or ulcer. Later, cancer may cause a rapidly growing, raised growth. Spread is first to the lymph nodes in one or both groin areas, and later to the nodes deep in the pelvic area. Distant spread via the blood is unusual.

### Risk Factors

Human papillomavirus infection is thought to be responsible for about 30% to 50% of vulvar cancers. Cigarette smoking and HIV infection also are associated with increased risk.

### Symptoms

A growth or lump on the vulva is the most common complaint, although some women may notice vulvar itching, pain, or bleeding. Up to 20% of patients have the disease discovered during a routine pelvic examination.

### Diagnosis

Cancer is usually suspected from a pelvic examination, but biopsy under local anesthesia using a skin punch that takes a small tissue sample is needed for a correct diagnosis.

### Determining Stage

A history taking and complete physical examination that includes careful pelvic and rectal examination are followed by a Pap test and examination of the cervix with a lighted magnifying instrument (colposcope). It may be necessary to examine the bladder outlet (urethra) and bladder by means of cystoscopy, and the anus and rectum using colonoscopy. X-rays of the chest and kidney are followed by CT or MRI of the pelvic area.

### Considerations

Both surgery and radiation have been effective, depending on the stage and location of the tumor. Improved techniques combining radiation therapy and drug therapy are needed to lessen the adverse effects of present-day treatment. Unlike cervical cancer that develops rather quickly from carcinoma in situ of the cervix, vulvar cancer appears to take many years to develop from in situ carcinoma. This long lag-period should enable women with preinvasive vulvar cancer to be diagnosed and treated before more serious, invasive cancer develops. The American Cancer Society includes pelvic examination in its recommendations for routine cancer-related checkups (*see* Appendix for Cancer Detection Guidelines).

*See also* Human Papillomavirus.

## WILMS' TUMOR

### Overview

Also known as nephroblastoma, this rare childhood kidney cancer occurs most often in children under 6 years old and accounts for about 6% of all pediatric cancers. Between 400 and 500 new cases are diagnosed each year in the United States. It usually affects only one kidney, but about 5% of Wilms' tumors are found in both kidneys. It is also more common among African Americans and among females. Wilms' tumor is of interest because it was the first malignant tumor successfully treated using combined surgery, radiation therapy, and chemotherapy, which today is standard therapy for many cancers. Present-day treatment cures more than 90% of patients with this disease.

### Type of Tumor and Spread

There are several varieties, all of which are remnants of the embryonic kidney (the kidney in the first several months following conception). The microscopic appearance of the tumor determines if it is a favorable or unfavorable type. The latter are fast growing varieties likely to metastasize (spread) at an early time and to be resistant to chemotherapy. Spread occurs from involvement or invasion of surrounding tissue, spread to adjacent lymph nodes, or dissemination through blood to lung and liver.

### Risk Factors

While there is a clear connection among Wilms' tumors, certain birth defect syndromes, and genetic deletions or mutations, most children with this type of cancer do not have any known birth defects or inherited gene changes. Only about 10% of Wilms' tumors have defects of the WT1 gene (Wilms' tumor suppressor gene). There is a strong link between Wilms' tumors and certain kinds of birth defects. About 15% of patients with Wilms' tumor also have birth defects.

### Symptoms

The most frequent is a painless mass in the abdomen or side below the ribs, most often discovered when the child is bathed. Approximately one-fourth of children have abdominal pain, fever, bloody urine, or high blood pressure.

### Diagnosis

A firm, rounded, mass or lump deep in the abdomen, usually on one side, is very suggestive of this cancer; and the disease is confirmed most often by abdominal CT.

### Determining Stage

Following a careful physical examination and urinalysis, blood tests are obtained to assess liver and kidney function. Imaging studies of the chest include x-rays and possibly CT.

### Considerations

Because Wilms' tumor is rare, few doctors except those in children's cancer centers have much experience in treating the disease. Treatment combining radiation therapy, chemotherapy, and surgery produces excellent results, with over 90% being cured. New medication and different doses of existing drugs are being evaluated to lessen adverse effects, and improve results in treating unfavorable tumors. Also, different treatment methods are being developed to improve the therapy of simultaneous cancer in both kidneys.

*See also* Childhood Cancer; Kidney Cancer (pages 173–174).

# Appendix

## CANCER DETECTION GUIDELINES

### Cancer-Related Checkup

A cancer-related checkup is recommended every 3 years for people aged 20–40 and every year for people age 40 and older. This exam should include health counseling, and depending on a person's age might include examinations for cancers of the thyroid, oral cavity, skin, lymph nodes, testes, and ovaries as well as for some nonmalignant diseases.

**Special tests for certain cancer sites are recommended as outlined below.**

### Breast

Women aged 40 and older should have an annual mammogram, an annual clinical breast examination (CBE) by a health care professional, and should perform monthly breast self-examination (BSE). The CBE should be conducted close to and preferably before the scheduled mammogram.

Women aged 20–39 should have a CBE by a health care professional every 3 years and should perform monthly BSE.

### Colon and Rectum

Beginning at age 50, men and women at average risk should follow one of these five testing schedules:

1) Fecal occult blood test (FOBT) every year*
2) Flexible sigmoidoscopy every 5 years**
3) FOBT every year and flexible sigmoidoscopy every 5 years*,**

*(Of the three options above, the American Cancer Society prefers option 3, annual FOBT and flexible sigmoidoscopy every 5 years)*

4) Double-contrast barium enema every 5 years
5) Colonoscopy every 10 years**

**For FOBT, the take-home multiple sample method should be used.*
***A digital rectal examination should be done at the same time as sigmoidoscopy or colonoscopy.*

**All positive test results should be followed up with colonoscopy.**

People should begin colorectal cancer screening earlier and/or undergo screening more often if they have any of the following colorectal cancer risk factors:

- A personal history of colorectal cancer or adenomatous polyps.
- A strong family history of colorectal cancer or polyps (cancer or polyps in a first-degree relative younger than 60 or in two first-degree relatives of any age); Note: a first-degree relative is defined as a parent, sibling, or child.
- A personal history of chronic inflammatory bowel disease.
- Families with hereditary colorectal cancer syndromes (familial adenomatous polyposis and hereditary nonpolyposis colon cancer).

**Prostate**

***Guideline Statement:*** Both prostate-specific antigen (PSA) and digital rectal examination (DRE) should be offered annually, beginning at age 50 years, to men who have at least a 10-year life expectancy. Men at high risk should begin testing at age 45 years. Information should be provided to men regarding potential risks and benefits of early detection and treatment of prostate cancer.

Men who choose to undergo testing should begin at age 50 years. However, men in high risk groups, such as African Americans and men who have a first-degree relative diagnosed with prostate cancer at a young age, should begin testing at 45 years. Note: a first-degree relative is defined as a father, brother, or son.

Men who ask their doctor to make the decision on their behalf should be tested. Discouraging testing is not appropriate. Also not offering testing is not appropriate.

Testing for prostate cancer in asymptomatic men can detect tumors at a more favorable stage (anatomic extent of disease). There has been a reduction in mortality from prostate cancer, but it has not been established that this is a direct result of screening.

An abnormal PSA test result has been defined as a value above 4.0 ng/ml. Some elevations in PSA may be due to benign conditions of the prostate.

The DRE of the prostate should be performed by health care workers skilled in recognizing subtle prostate abnormalities, including those of symmetry and consistency, as well as the more classic findings of marked induration or nodules. DRE is less effective in detecting prostate carcinoma compared with PSA.

**Uterus**

***Cervix:*** Pap test and pelvic examination for women who are or have been sexually active or have reached age 18, every year; after 3 or more consecutive satisfactory normal annual exams, the Pap test may be performed less frequently at the discretion of the physician.

***Endometrium:*** For women with or at high risk for hereditary nonpolyposis colon cancer (HNPCC), annual screening should be offered for endometrial cancer with endometrial biopsy beginning at age 35.

### Reference

American Cancer Society. *Cancer Facts and Figures 2001.* Atlanta, GA.

# Resources

## AMERICAN CANCER SOCIETY RESOURCES

The American Cancer Society (ACS) provides educational materials and information on cancer, offers a variety of patient programs, and directs people to services in their community. To find your local office, contact us at 800-ACS-2345 or visit our web site *(http://www.cancer.org).*

National Home Office
1599 Clifton Road NE
Atlanta, GA 30329-4251
Toll-Free: 800-ACS-2345 (800-227-2345)
Web site: *http://www.cancer.org*

### American Cancer Society Programs and Services

*The ACS programs and services listed below may be of special interest to those with cancer and their loved ones. Contact the American Cancer Society for more information about services in your area.*

#### Cancer Survivors' Network

This network provides both a telephone-based and an on-line community that welcome cancer survivors, friends, and families to share and communicate with others with similar interests and experiences. The program offers a vibrant community of real people supporting one another and sharing personal experiences with cancer. The web site enables registered members to have live, private chats, to create personal web pages to share experiences, thoughts, and wisdom, to help people create personal support communities of people who share common concerns and interests, and offers information about resources. The telephone component uses an interactive voice response system and consists of prerecorded discussions among survivors and family. Users can navigate from discussion to discussion or leave a comment or question 24 hours a day, 7 days a week, at 877-333-HOPE (877-333-4673).

#### Hope Lodges

Hope Lodges are temporary residential facilities providing sleeping rooms and related facilities for people with cancer who are undergoing outpatient treatment and their family members. Approval from a doctor or referring agency is necessary.

### I Can Cope

This program addresses the educational and psychological needs of people with cancer and their families. A series of eight classes discusses the disease, coping with daily health problems, controlling cancer-related pain, nutrition for the person with cancer, expressing feelings, living with limitations, and local resources. Through lectures, group discussions, and study assignments, the course helps people with cancer regain a sense of control over their lives.

> *Taking Charge of Money Matters.* This is an ACS workshop offered through the I Can Cope program. This workshop offers financial guidance for cancer survivors and their families. Topics include the fundamentals of insurance, estate planning, returning to work, disability insurance, how to improve your financial planning, financial resources, and how to create a budget. Call the ACS for more information.

### Look Good...Feel Better

Toll-Free: 800-395-LOOK (800-395-6005)

Founded in partnership with the National Cosmetology Association and the Cosmetic, Toiletry, and Fragrance Association (CTFA) Foundation as a free national public service program dedicated to teaching women with cancer how to restore a healthy appearance and self-image during and after chemotherapy and radiation therapy.

### Man to Man

This program provides accurate, factual information to men and their partners about prostate cancer in a supportive environment following essential guidelines that assure program integrity and credibility. Man to Man is an ideal vehicle by which new relationships are formed between patients/survivors and care providers with a two-way exchange of information, trust, and respect.

### Reach to Recovery

This program is designed to help patients with breast cancer cope with their diagnosis, treatment, and recovery. The volunteers for this program are women who have had breast cancer and are specially trained to share their knowledge and experiences in a supportive and nonintrusive manner. Ongoing support groups are available to help deal with the challenges of breast cancer. Reach to Recovery also provides early support to women who may have breast cancer or have just been diagnosed with cancer.

## OTHER ORGANIZATIONS

Listings in this section represent organizations that operate on a national level and provide some type of service or resource to consumers related to cancer. This list is designed to offer a starting point for seeking information, support, and needed resources. Most of the organizations listed here can be contacted via phone, fax, or e-mail, and some through their web site. Many of the web sites provide much of the same information that is available by postal mail. Some organizations are solely web-based and will require Internet access. Keep in mind that new web sites appear daily while old ones expand, move, or disappear entirely. Some of the web sites or content outlined below may change. Often, a simple Internet search will point to the new web site for a given organization. The American Cancer Society web site provides links to outside sources of cancer information as well (*http://www.cancer.org*).

There is a vast amount of information about cancer on the Internet. This information can be very valuable to those facing cancer in making decisions about their illness and treatment. However, since any group of individuals can publish on the Internet, it is important to consider the credentials and reputation of the organization providing information. Internet information should not be a substitute for medical advice.

The agencies, organizations, corporations, and publications represented in this resource guide are not necessarily endorsed by the American Cancer Society. This guide is provided for assistance in obtaining information only.

### Cancer and Health Information

*The listings in this section include resources for general and specific information about cancer and cancer-related health concerns and conditions. Contact the ACS for additional resources, including resources for specific cancer types.*

#### AARP

601 E Street NW
Washington, DC 20049
Toll-Free: 800-424-3410
E-mail: member@aarp.org
Web site: *http://www.aarp.org*
Web site (for Pharmacy Service): *http://www.aarppharmacy.com*

This organization offers membership to anyone over age 50 for a small yearly fee. It focuses on addressing the needs of older people on a national level. The web site includes information on a member pharmacy service that offers discounts on drugs.

**AIDS Clinical Trials Information Service (ACTIS)**

PO Box 6421
Rockville, MD 20849-6421
Toll-Free: 800-TRIALS-A (800-874-2572)
Toll-Free (TTY): 888-480-3739
Phone: 301-519-0459
Fax: 301-519-6616
E-mail: ACTIS@actis.org
Web site: *http://www.actis.org*

The ACTIS is federally supported and sponsored. It provides up-to-date information about clinical trials that evaluate experimental drugs and other therapies for HIV infection and AIDS-related conditions.

**AMC Cancer Research Center & Foundation**

1600 Pierce Street
Denver, CO 80214
Toll-Free: 800-321-1557
Toll-Free (Counseling): 800-525-3777
Phone: 303-233-6501
Web site: *http://www.amc.org*

Through the counseling line of this nonprofit research center, you can request free publications and receive answers to questions about cancer. The web site contains an area about ongoing research and general information about specific types of cancer.

**American Brain Tumor Association**

2720 River Road
Des Plaines, IL 60018
Phone: 847-827-9910
Fax: 847-827-9918
E-mail: info@abta.org
Web site: *http://www.abta.org*

Offers publications and services to people with brain tumors and their families, including information about treatments, coping mechanisms, support resources, research updates, a pen pal program, and a section for kids.

**American Institute for Cancer Research (AICR)**

1759 R Street NW
Washington, DC 20009
Toll-Free: 800-843-8114

Phone: 202-328-7744
e-mail: aicrweb@aicr.org
Web site: *http://www.aicr.org*

Focuses on the relationship between diet and nutrition and cancer prevention and treatment. Creates public health education programs, funds research, and provides information to the public and health care professionals.

**American Medical Association (AMA)**
515 North State Street
Chicago, IL 60610
Phone: 312-464-5000
Web site: *http://www.ama-assn.org*

The AMA develops and promotes standards in medical practice, research, and education. Under the consumer health information section, the web site contains databases on doctors and hospitals, which can be searched by medical specialty. A pull-down menu of specific conditions (such as breast cancer) is also provided.

**American Society of Clinical Oncology (ASCO)**
1900 Duke Street, Suite 200
Alexandria, VA 22314
Phone: 703-299-0150
Fax: 703-299-1044
E-mail: asco@asco.org
Web site: *http://www.asco.org*

An international medical society representing about 10,000 cancer specialists involved in clinical research and patient care. The web site is a resource for cancer patients, doctors, and researchers and includes patient guides, a glossary of cancer terms, an ASCO member oncologist locator, news and information about different cancers and drug treatments, information about cancer legislation, summaries of government reports, and links to related sites.

**The American Society for Therapeutic Radiology and Oncology (ASTRO)**
12500 Fair Lakes Circle, Suite 375
Fairfax, VA 22033-3882
Toll-Free: 800-962-7876
Phone: 703-227-0187
Fax: 703-502-7852
Web site: *http://www.astro.org*

Focusing on the use of radiation therapy for the treatment of cancer, this society's web site includes an overview of radiation therapy and a list of frequently asked questions. Some breast cancer–specific information is also available.

**Association of Community Cancer Centers (ACCC)**

11600 Nebel Street, Suite 201
Rockville, MD 20852
Phone: 301-984-9496
Fax: 301-770-1949
Web site: *http://www.accc-cancer.org*

This national organization includes over 650 hospitals, cancer centers, group practices, and free-standing clinics. This web site contains a searchable database of cancer centers listed by state as well as information about oncology drugs (registration is required) and specific cancers.

**Breast Cancer Awareness**

US Department of Defense
Web site: *http://www.tricaresw.af.mil/breastcd/index.html*

An interactive web site provides information about breast cancer diagnosis and treatment. The site contains detailed downloadable text on breast cancer as well as movies illustrating some of the steps involved in detection and treatment.

**Canadian Cancer Society (CCS)**

10 Alcorn Avenue, Suite 200
Toronto, Ontario M4V 3B1
Phone: 416-961-7223
Fax: 416-961-4189
E-mail: info@cis.cancer.ca
Web site: *http://www.cancer.ca*

This organization provides facts about cancer, treatment, prevention, and Canadian units of the CCS in English and French.

**CancerGuide**

E-mail: steve.dunn@cancerguide.org
Web site: *http://cancerguide.org*

Information about cancer assembled by a computer-literate layperson: cancer fundamentals, recommended books, clinical trials, how to research medical literature, and alternative therapies.

**Cancer Research Institute (CRI)**

681 Fifth Avenue
New York, NY 10022
Toll-Free: 800-99-CANCER (800-992-6237)
Phone: 212-688-7515
E-mail: info@cancerresearch.org
Web site: *http://www.cancerresearch.org*

An institute funding cancer research and providing public information on cancer immunology and cancer treatment, the CRI helps locate immunotherapy clinical trials, and offers a cancer reference guide and other informational booklets.

**Centers for Disease Control and Prevention (CDC)**

Cancer Prevention and Control Program
CDC/DCPC
4770 Buford Highway NE
MS K64
Atlanta, GA 30341
Toll-Free: 888-842-6355
Fax: 770-488-4760
E-mail: cancerinfo@cdc.gov
Web site: *http://www.cdc.gov/cancer*

The CDC is an agency of the United States Department of Health and Human Services. Their mission is to promote health and quality of life by preventing and controlling disease, injury, and disability. The CDC provides information about chronic diseases such as cancer. The web site contains a searchable map of centers, information about cancer, downloadable publications, and links to related sources. *Spanish-speaking staff and Spanish materials are available.*

**Environmental Protection Agency (EPA)**

Ariel Rios Building
1200 Pennsylvania Avenue NW
Washington, DC 20460
Phone: 202-260-2090
Web site: *http://www.epa.gov*

The EPA implements the federal laws designed to promote public health by protecting our nation's air, water, and soil from harmful pollution. The web site offers environmental news, community concerns, information about laws and other regulations, and links to other sources of information.

**HealthScout**

Web site: *http://www.healthscout.com*

Healthscout is a general health web site that provides health care news and medical information. It also provides connections to other health resources.

**International Agency for Research on Cancer (IARC)**

World Health Organization
150 cours Albert Thomas
F-69372 Lyon cedex 08, France
Phone: 33-4-72-73-84-85
Fax: 33-4-72-73-85-75
Web site: *http://www.iarc.fr*

IARC coordinates and conducts research on the causes of human cancer and the mechanisms of carcinogenesis. The *IARC Monographs,* available on the IARC web site, are critical reviews and evaluations of evidence on the carcinogenicity of a wide range of human exposures. The IARC web site contains three databases with information on the occurrence of cancer worldwide, a database including carcinogenic risks to humans, a list of publications, and links to related cancer sites.

**International Association of Laryngectomees**

8900 Thornton Road
PO Box 99311
Stockton, CA 95209
Toll-Free: 866-IAL-FORU (866-425-3678)
Fax: 209-472-0516
Web site: *http://www.larynxlink.com*

This voluntary organization is dedicated to the total rehabilitation of laryngectomees. Promotes exchange and dissemination of ideas and information to laryngectomee clubs and to the public.

**International Myeloma Foundation**

12650 Riverside Drive, Suite 206
North Hollywood, CA 91607
Toll-Free: 800-452-CURE (800-452-2873)
Phone: 818-487-7455
Fax: 818-487-7454
E-mail: TheIMF@myeloma.org
Web site: *http://www.myeloma.org*

Dedicated to improving quality of life for myeloma patients, while working toward prevention and a cure.

**Let's Face It USA**

PO Box 29972
Bellingham, WA 98228-1972
Phone: 360-676-7325
E-mail: letsfaceit@faceit.org
Web site: *http://www.faceit.org*

Information and support network for people with head and neck cancer and others with facial disfigurement.

**Leukemia & Lymphoma Society, Inc.**

1311 Mamaroneck Avenue
White Plains, NY 10605
Toll-Free: 800-955-4572
Phone: 914-949-5213
Web site: *http://www.leukemia.org*

This national voluntary health agency, which was formerly known as the Leukemia Society of America, offers a variety of service programs and resources related to leukemia, lymphoma, Hodgkin's disease, and myeloma, including improving quality of life. Contact the national office for a listing of local chapters.

**Lymphoma Research Foundation of America**

8800 Venice Boulevard, Suite 207
Los Angeles, CA 90034
Phone: 310-204-7040
Fax: 310-204-7043
Web site: *http://www.lymphoma.org*

Funds medical research devoted to improving lymphoma treatments, and offers a newsletter and support system to patients and their families.

**MayoClinic.com**

Web site: *http://www.mayohealth.org*

This web site contains a database searchable by keyword and topic. It also offers a question and answer link to a doctor at the Mayo Clinic, as well as links to reference articles and cancer organizations.

**Medscape**

Web site: *http://www.medscape.com*

Although registration is required to view some of the content, this web site offers a great deal of information on prescription drugs as well as medical articles. There are also links to several organizations, cancer centers, database and education web sites, journals, and government sites. The web site is also searchable by key word. Registration is free.

**MedWatch**

Toll-Free: 800-332-1088
Web site: *http://www.fda.gov/medwatch*

Through MedWatch, the FDA maintains an adverse event and product reporting program. The organization accepts reports of problems with food, drugs, or devices from the general public. The web site includes medical product safety alerts as well as searchable FDA safety databases and FDA medical bulletins.

**National Alliance of Breast Cancer Organizations (NABCO)**

9 East Thirty-Seventh Street, Tenth Floor
New York, NY 10016
Toll-Free: 888-80-NABCO (888-806-2226)
Phone (emergencies only): 212-889-0606
Fax: 212-689-1213
E-mail: nabcoinfo@aol.com
Web site: *http://www.nabco.org*

This nonprofit organization includes a network of more than 400 organizations. The NABCO web site includes information about breast cancer and breast health, a directory of nationwide events, a resource list, a list of local support groups, and a directory of clinical trials. The site also allows women to register for a mammography e-mail reminder.

**National Brain Tumor Foundation**

414 Thirteenth Street, Suite 700
Oakland, CA 94612-2603
Toll-Free: 800-934-CURE (800-934-2873)
Phone: 510-839-9777
Fax: 510-839-9779
E-mail: nbtf@braintumor.org
Web site: *http://www.braintumor.org*

Raises funds for research and provides information and support services to people with brain tumors and their families.

**The National Breast Cancer Coalition**

1707 L Street NW, Suite 1060
Washington, DC 20036
Toll-Free: 800-622-2838
Phone: 202-296-7477
Fax: 202-265-6854
Web site: *http://www.natlbcc.org*

Strives to involve women with breast cancer and those that care about them in changing public policy. Goals include increasing breast cancer research funding and improving access to screening, increasing the influence that breast cancer survivors have over research, clinical trials, and national policy.

**National Cancer Institute (NCI)**

NCI Public Inquiries Office
Building 31, Room 10A31
31 Center Drive, MSC 2580
Bethesda, MD 20892-2580
Toll-Free: 800-4-CANCER (800-422-6237)
Web site: *http://www.cancer.gov*

This US government agency provides information on cancer research, diagnosis, and treatment through several services (see list below). People with cancer, caregivers, and health care professionals may call the NCI's toll-free telephone service for cancer-related information. *Spanish-speaking staff and Spanish materials are available.*

*For more information about or area listings of Community Clinical Oncology Programs, Comprehensive Cancer Centers, or Clinical Cancer Centers, call NCI at 800-4-CANCER. Or go to* http://cis.nci.nih.gov/fact/nci.htm *and choose* Community Clinical Oncology Program *or* The National Cancer Institute Cancer Centers Program.

*See also listings for NCI's CancerTrials and Clinical Trials Cooperative Group Program, in the* Clinical Trials *section (pages 237–238).*

***CancerFax***

Toll-Free Fax: 800-624-2511
Fax: 301-402-5874

CancerFax includes information about cancer treatment, screening, prevention, and supportive care. To obtain a contents list, dial the fax number from a fax machine hand set and follow the recorded instructions.

***Cancer Information Service (CIS)***

Toll-Free: 800-4-CANCER (800-422-6237)
Toll-Free (TTY): 800-332-8615
Web site: *http://cis.nci.nih.gov*

The CIS provides information to consumers and health care professionals. Call CIS for a referral to a pain control clinic or support group in your area. The web site contains a wealth of information including pamphlets and brochures on cancer diagnosis, treatment, research, and prevention. *Spanish-speaking staff is available.*

***CANCERLIT (Bibliographic Database)***

Web site: *http://cnetdb.nci.nih.gov/cancerlit.html*

This searchable site is maintained by the NCI and contains cancer and pain articles published in medical and scientific journals, books, government reports, and articles that were presented at national meetings. A link to the PDQ (CancerNet/NCI database) search engine is provided which allows you to search for clinical trials by state, city, and type of cancer.

***CancerNet***

Web site: *http://cancernet.gov*
Web site (Spanish version): *http://cancernet.gov/sp_menu.htm*
Web site (On-line ordering): *http://publications.nci.nih.gov*

A comprehensive web site that contains information on diagnosis, treatment, support, resources, literature, clinical trials, prevention and risk factors, and testing. Up to twenty publications can be ordered on-line. The publications list is searchable. *Some publications are available in Spanish.*

**National Center for Complementary and Alternative Medicine (NCCAM)**

National Institutes of Health
NCCAM Clearinghouse
PO Box 8218
Silver Spring, MD 20907-8218
Toll-Free: 888-644-6226
Phone outside the US: 301-231-7537, ext. 5
Fax: 301-495-4957
Web site: *http://nccam.nih.gov*

This site provides information on complementary and alternative methods being promoted to treat different diseases.

**National Comprehensive Cancer Network (NCCN)**

50 Huntingdon Pike, Suite 200
Rockledge, PA 19046
Toll-Free: 888-909-NCCN (800-909-6226)
Phone: 215-728-4788
Fax: 215-728-3877
E-mail: information@nccn.org
Web site: *http://www.nccn.org*

The NCCN is a nonprofit organization that is an alliance of cancer centers. The American Cancer Society has partnered with NCCN to translate the NCCN Clinical Practice Guidelines into patient-friendly resources. The Clinical Practice Guidelines are available to doctors by contacting NCCN. The *Treatment Guidelines for Patients,* which are available on-line, offer the latest information for a variety of cancers and cancer-related conditions (e.g., breast cancer, prostate cancer, colon and rectal cancer, pain control, nausea and vomiting). The guidelines offer easy to understand information for patients and family members about treatment options, and printed copies of the guidelines are available through the ACS.

**National Consumers League**

1701 K Street NW, Suite 1201
Washington, DC 20006
Phone: 202-835-3323
Fax: 202-835-0747
Web site: *http://www.nclnet.org*

Experts in law, business, and labor provide consumer protection and advocacy. Publishes education brochures about general health issues, including cancer screening tests.

**National Council Against Health Fraud**

PO Box 141
Fort Lee, NJ 07024
Phone: 201-723-2955
E-mail: ncahf@worldnet.att.net
Web site: *http://www.ncahf.org*

Focuses on health misinformation, fraud, and quackery, and provides information on unusual methods of cancer management. Can refer people to lawyers and help those who have had negative experiences to share their story.

**National Institutes of Health (NIH)**

Bethesda, MD 20892
Phone: 301-496-4000
E-mail (please submit questions and requests via e-mail):
nihinfo@od.nih.gov
Web site: *http://www.nih.gov*

The NIH is an agency of the Public Health Services, which in turn is part of the US Department of Health and Human Services. The NIH mission is to uncover new knowledge that will lead to better health for everyone. NIH conducts research in its own laboratories, supports the research of non-Federal scientists, helps in the training of research investigators, and fosters communication of medical information.

***National Institutes of Health Consensus Program***

PO Box 2577
Kensington, MD 20891
Toll-Free: 800-644-2667
E-mail: consensus@od.nih.gov
Web site: *http://consensus.nih.gov*

Updates practicing doctors and the public with current responsible information on the pros and cons of various medical technologies.

***US National Library of Medicine***

National Institutes of Health
Department of Health and Human Services
8600 Rockville Pike
Bethesda, MD 20894
Web site: *http://www.nlm.nih.gov*

Provides a search engine for health, medical, scientific literature, and research as well as links to other government resources.

*Internet Grateful Med*

Web site: *http://igm.nlm.nih.gov*

Provides access to millions of literature references and abstracts in Medline and other databases, with links to on-line journals. The site is searchable by key words.

*NLM Gateway*

Web site: *http://gateway.nlm.nih.gov/gw/Cmd*

Offers links to searchable databases and allows users to search simultaneously in multiple retrieval systems.

*PubMed*

Web site: *http://www.ncbi.nlm.nih.gov/PubMed*

Provides access to millions of literature references and abstracts in Medline and other databases, with links to on-line journals. The site is searchable by key word.

**National Kidney Cancer Association**

1234 Sherman Avenue, Suite 203
Evanston, IL 60202-1375
Toll-Free: 800-850-9132
Phone: 847-332-1051
Fax: 847-332-2978
E-mail: office@kidneycancerassociation.org
Web site: *http://www.nkca.org*

Provides information to patients and doctors, sponsors research on kidney cancer, gives referrals to doctors, publishes a newsletter, and acts as a patient advocate.

**National Lymphedema Network (NLN)**

Latham Square
1611 Telegraph Avenue, Suite 1111
Oakland, CA 94612
Toll-Free (Hotline): 800-541-3259
Phone: 510-208-3200
Fax: 510-208-3110
Web site: *http://www.lymphnet.org*

The web site for this nonprofit agency offers information about lymphedema, a referral service to medical and therapeutic treatment centers, and information on locating or establishing local support groups. It publishes a newsletter, which contains articles about lymphedema and a resource guide of treatment centers, doctors, therapists, and suppliers.

**National Toxicology Program (NTP)**

National Institutes of Health
National Institute of Environmental Health Sciences
Durham, NC 27704
Web site: *http://ntp-server.niehs.nih.gov*

The NTP's *Report on Carcinogens* identifies substances and mixtures or exposure circumstances that are "known" or are "reasonably anticipated" to cause cancer, and to which a significant number of Americans are exposed. The *Report on Carcinogens* is published every two years and is available on the NTP web site.

**National Women's Health Information Center**

The Office on Women's Health
US Department of Health and Human Services
8550 Arlington Boulevard, Suite 300
Fairfax, VA 22031
Toll-Free: 800-994-WOMAN (800-994-9662)
Toll-Free (TDD): 888-220-5546
Web site: *http://www.4woman.gov*
Web site (Spanish version): *http://www.4woman.gov/Spanish/index.htm*

This web site has a searchable database of information on various women's health issues, including breast cancer. Documents accessible through this site include information from the NCI, the CDC, and several other government agencies. The site contains a section for special groups, which separates breast cancer and other health information by specific minority group. It also contains links to on-line medical dictionaries and journals.

**OncoLink**

University of Pennsylvania Cancer Center
E-mail: editors@oncolink.upenn.edu
Web site: *http://www.oncolink.com*

Sponsored by the University of Pennsylvania Cancer Center Resource, this web site provides information on cancer, including clinical trials, support groups, educational materials, cancer screening and prevention, financial questions, and other resources for people with cancer.

**Physicians Data Query (PDQ)**

National Cancer Institute
Toll-Free: 800-4-CANCER (800-422-6237)
Web site: *http://cancernet.nci.nih.gov/pdqfull.html*

Computerized listing of up-to-date and accurate information for people with cancer and health care professionals on the latest treatments, research studies, and clinical trials.

**Quackwatch**

Web site: *http://www.quackwatch.com*

Quackwatch, Inc. is a nonprofit corporation whose purpose is to combat health-related frauds, myths, fads, and fallacies. The Quackwatch web site is a comprehensive source of information regarding fraudulent claims. *Information is offered in German, Spanish, French, and Portuguese, as well as in English.*

**Skin Cancer Foundation**

245 Fifth Avenue, Suite 1403
New York, NY 10016
Toll-Free: 800-SKIN-490 (800-754-6490)
Fax: 212-725-5751
E-mail: info@skincancer.org
Web site: *http://www.skincancer.org*

Conducts educational programs for the public and medical communities; supports medical training, cancer screening, and prevention programs; provides information about safe sun exposure for children and adults; and publishes a journal.

**The Susan G. Komen Breast Cancer Foundation**

5005 LBJ Freeway, Suite 250
Dallas, TX 75244
Toll-Free (Breast Care Helpline): 800-IM-AWARE (800-462-9273)
Phone: 972-855-1600
Fax: 972-855-1605
E-mail: helpline@komen.org
Web site: *http://www.komen.org*

This organization promotes research, education, screening, and treatment. The web site contains the latest news and information regarding breast health, drug therapies, treatment options, educational events and meetings, survivor stories, and other breast cancer–related information.

**United Ostomy Association**

19772 MacArthur Boulevard, Suite 200
Irvine, CA 92612
Toll-Free: 800-826-0826
Web site: *http://www.uoa.org*

This volunteer-based health organization provides education, information, support, and advocacy for people who have had or will have intestinal or urinary diversions.

**US TOO! International, Inc.**

5003 Fairview Avenue
Downers Grove, IL 60515
Toll-Free: 800-80-US-TOO (800-808-7866)
Phone: 630-795-1002
Fax: 630-795-1602
E-mail: ustoo@ustoo.com
Web site: *http://www.ustoo.com*

This independent group provides prostate cancer survivors and their families with emotional and educational support.

**Y-ME National Breast Cancer Organization**

212 West Van Buren, Suite 500
Chicago, IL 60607
Toll-Free Hotline: 800-221-2141
Toll-Free Hotline (Spanish): 800-986-9505
Phone: 312-986-8338
Fax: 312-294-8597
Web site: *http://www.y-me.org*
Web site (Spanish version): *http://www.y-me.org/spanish.htm*

This organization focuses on providing information and support to people with breast cancer and their families. Y-ME provides a national hotline, public meetings and seminars, workshops for professionals, referral services, support groups, a newsletter, a resource library, a teen program, and advocacy information.

### Children's Cancers

*The listings in this section include resources for children with cancer. (Note: The majority of children with cancer are treated at large pediatric cancer centers in clinical trials of the Children's Oncology Group. For information about this group, see* Clinical Trials, pages 237–238.*) Contact ACS for a list of children's cancer camps in the United States.*

**Candlelighters Childhood Cancer Foundation**

3910 Warner Street
Kensington, MD 20895
Toll-Free: 800-366-2233
Phone: 301-962-3520
Fax: 301-962-3521
E-mail: info@candlelighters.org
Web site: *http://www.candlelighters.org*

Provides information, support, and advocacy to families of children with cancer, survivors of childhood cancer, and professionals who work with them.

**Chai Lifeline/Camp Simcha**

151 West Thirtieth Street
New York, NY 10001
Toll-Free: 877-CHAI-LIFE (877-242-4543)
Phone: 212-465-1301
Fax: 212-465-0949
Web site: *http://www.chailifeline.org*

Provides a kosher camp for children with cancer or hematological conditions, free of charge, including transportation from anywhere in the world. Open to children of any religion who meet the medical approval of the director.

**Children's Hospice International**

901 North Pitt Street, Suite 230
Alexandria, VA 22314
Toll-Free: 800-24-CHILD (800-242-4453)
Phone: 703-684-0330
Fax: 703-684-0226
Web site: *http://www.chionline.org*

Creates hospice support for children and provides medical and technical assistance, research, and education to their families and health care professionals.

**Children's Oncology Camping Association International**

PO Box 35
Mountain Center, CA 92561
Toll-Free: 800-737-2667
Web site: *http://www.coca-intl.org*

Provides international directory of oncology camps.

**The Children's Organ Transplant Association (COTA)**

2501 COTA Drive
Bloomington, IN 47403
Toll-Free: 800-366-2682
E-mail: jennifer@cota.org
Web site: *http://www.cota.org*

Helps families and communities raise funds for children needing transplants and transplant-related expenses.

**Federation for Children with Special Needs**

1135 Tremont Street, Suite 420
Boston, MA 02120
Toll-Free in MA: 800-331-0688
Phone: 617-236-7210
Fax: 617-572-2094
E-mail: fcsninfo@fcsn.org
Web site: *http://www.fcsn.org*

This information and referral agency provides training for parents on understanding their rights under special education laws, and helping parents become health care advocates.

**Make-A-Wish Foundation of America**

3550 North Central Avenue, Suite 300
Phoenix, AZ 85012
Toll-Free: 800-722-WISH (800-722-9474)
Phone: 602-279-WISH (602-279-9474)
Fax: 602-279-0855
E-mail: mawfa@wish.org
Web site: *http://www.wish.org*

This organization grants wishes to children between the ages of 2 and 18 who have life-threatening illnesses.

**Ronald McDonald House Charities**

1 Kroc Drive
Oak Brook, IL 60523
Web site: *http://www.rmhc.com*

Supports temporary lodging facilities for the families of seriously ill children being treated at nearby hospitals.

**Starlight Children's Foundation**

5900 Wilshire Boulevard, Suite 2530
Los Angeles, CA 90036
Phone: 323-634-0080
E-mail: info@starlight.org
Web site: *http://www.starlight.org*

Provides entertainment and recreational activities for seriously ill children ages 4–18 through mobile "fun centers," PC Pal computers, hospital events, and wish-granting activities in chapter areas.

**The Sunshine Foundation**

1041 Mill Creek Drive
Feasterville, PA 19053
Phone: 215-396-4770
Fax: 215-396-4774
Web site: *http://www.sunshinefoundation.org*

Grants wishes to chronically or terminally ill and handicapped children whose families are under a financial strain due to their child's illness.

**The Sunshine Kids**

2814 Virginia
Houston, TX 77098
Toll-Free: 800-594-5756
Web site: *http://www.sunshinekids.org*

Offers sports, cultural events, and group activities, free of charge, to children receiving cancer treatment.

**Wigs for Kids**

Executive Club Building
21330 Center Ridge Road, Suite C
Rocky River, OH 44116
Phone: 440-333-4433
Fax: 440-333-0200
E-mail: info@wigsforkids.org
Web site: *http://www.wigsforkids.org*

Wigs for Kids is a nonprofit organization providing hair replacement solutions for children affected by hair loss due to chemotherapy, radiation therapy, alopecia, burns, or other medical conditions.

## Clinical Trials

*The organizations listed in this section may help you understand clinical trials, identify ongoing clinical trials, or explore the findings of closed clinical trials.*

**CancerTrials**

National Cancer Institute
Web site: *http://cancertrials.nci.nih.gov*

This site offers information about ongoing cancer clinical trials and explanations of what a trial is and what is involved. A link to the PDQ (CancerNet/NCI database) search engine allows you to search for clinical trials by state, city, and type of cancer.

*Clinical Trials and Insurance Coverage: A Resource Guide*
Web site: *http://cancertrials.nci.nih.gov/understanding/indepth/insurance/index.html*

Part of the NCI's CancerTrials web site, this site offers information regarding the cost of clinical trials and how to determine if you will be covered under your health plan. Information about financial assistance programs for the needy is also available.

**Children's Oncology Group (COG)**
440 East Huntington Drive
PO Box 60012
Arcadia, CA 91066-6012
Toll-Free: 800-458-NCCF (800-458-6223)
Fax: 626-447-6359
Web site: *http://www.nccf.org*

This international collaborative group develops protocols, conducts clinical trials, and reviews treatment results. Member institutions are located in almost every state and province at over 235 medical centers. The group is affiliated with the National Childhood Cancer Foundation, which runs all fundraising for COG.

**ClinicalTrials.gov**
US National Institutes of Health
National Library of Medicine
Web site: *http://clinicaltrials.gov/ct/gui/c/r*

ClinicalTrials.gov provides current information about clinical research studies.

**Clinical Trials Cooperative Group Program**
National Cancer Institute
Web site: *http://cis.nci.nih.gov/fact/1_4.htm*

This program promotes and supports clinical trials of new cancer treatments. The cooperative groups are composed of academic institutions and cancer treatment centers throughout the United States, Canada, and Europe.

### Family Support

**Cancer Family Care**
2421 Auburn Avenue
Cincinnati, OH 45219
Phone: 513-731-3346
Fax: 513-458-3582
Web site: *http://www.cancerfamilycare.org*

A nonprofit psychosocial counseling agency for people with cancer and their families in Ohio and Kentucky.

**Centering Corporation**

PO Box 4600
Omaha, NE 68104
Phone: 402-553-1200
Fax: 402-553-0507
E-mail: center@centering.org
Web site: *http://www.centering.org*

This group offers resources for bereavement and coping with loss and sells over 100 books for children and adults.

**The Compassionate Friends**

PO Box 3696
Oakbrook, IL 60522-3696
Toll-Free: 877-969-0010
Phone: 630-990-0010
Fax: 630-990-0246
E-mail: marion@compassionatefriends.org
Web site: *http://www.compassionatefriends.org*

This nonprofit organization's nationwide and international chapters offer support for bereaved parents and siblings.

**GriefNet**

Web site: *http://griefnet.org*

This nonprofit site offers support for people dealing with grief, death, and major loss. Links to a companion site where children and parents can pose questions and concerns.

**National Association of Hospital Hospitality Houses, Inc.**

PO Box 18087
Asheville, NC 28814-0087
Toll-Free: 800-542-9730
Phone: 828-253-1188
Fax: 828-253-8082
E-mail: helpinghomes@nahhh.org
Web site: *http://www.nahhh.org*

Membership organization of facilities that coordinate lodging and accommodations for people receiving medical care.

**National Family Caregivers Association**

10400 Connecticut Avenue, #500
Kensington, MD 20895-3944
Toll-Free: 800-896-3650
Fax: 301-942-2302
E-mail: info@nfcacares.org
Web site: *http://www.nfcacares.org*

Provides research, education, support, advocacy, and respite care to caregivers.

**Ronald McDonald House Charities**

1 Kroc Drive
Oak Brook, IL 60523
Web site: *http://www.rmhc.com*

Supports temporary lodging facilities for the families of seriously ill children being treated at nearby hospitals.

**VHL Family Alliance**

171 Clinton Road
Brookline, MA 02445-5815
Toll-Free: 800-767-4VHL (800-767-4845)
Phone: 617-277-5667
Fax: 617-734-8233
E-mail: info@vhl.org
Web site: *http://www.vhl.org*

Provides literature and information, referrals, and research resources to von Hippel-Lindau (VHL) syndrome patients and their families.

**Well Spouse Foundation**

30 East Fortieth Street PH
New York, NY 10016
Toll-Free: 800-838-0879
Phone: 212-685-8815
Fax: 212-685-8676
Web site: *http://www.wellspouse.org*

Offers support to husbands, wives, and partners of people who are chronically ill and/or disabled.

## Home Health Care

**Amherst H. Wilder Foundation**

919 Lafond Avenue
St. Paul, MN 55104-2198
Phone: 651-642-4000
Web site: *http://www.wilder.org*

Offers services such as psychiatric clinics for children and the elderly, community services, and senior housing.

**Gentiva Health Services**

3 Huntington Quadrangle, 2S
Melville, NY 11747-8943
Toll-Free: 888-GENTIVA (888-436-8482)
Web site: *http://www.gentiva.com*

Provides community home health care services, including the coordination of health care services, home medical equipment, and infusion therapy. Professionals specialize in areas such as physical therapy, speech pathology, pediatric and geriatric care, and general nursing services.

**Home Care Guide for Advanced Cancer**

American College of Physicians-
American Society of Internal Medicine (ACP-ASIM)
190 North Independence Mall West
Philadelphia, PA 19106-1572
Toll-Free: 800-523-1546, x2600
Phone: 215-351-2600
E-mail: custserv@mail.acponline.com
Web site: *http://www.acponline.org/public/h_care/index.html*

The ACP-ASIM offers this free online book to help caregivers deal with the complex issues involved in caring for a person with cancer. The entire contents of the book can be downloaded.

**National Association for Home Care**

228 Seventh Street SE
Washington, DC 20003
Phone: 202-547-7424
Fax: 202-547-3540
Web site: *http://www.nahc.org*

The NAHC provides a state-by-state database of phone numbers for home care and hospice agencies.

**Oley Foundation**

214 Hun Memorial, A-28
Albany Medical Center
Albany, NY 12208-3478
Toll-Free: 800-776-OLEY (800-776-6539)
Phone: 518-262-5079
Fax: 518-262-5528
E-mail: bishopj@mail.amc.edu
Web site: *http://www.wizvax.net/oleyfdn*

Support for home parenteral and/or enteral nutrition therapy through a newsletter, conferences, meetings, and outreach activities.

**Visiting Nurse Associations of America**

11 Beacon Street, Suite 910
Boston, MA 02108
Phone: 617-523-4042
Fax: 617-227-4843
Web site: *http://www.vnaa.org*

This organization's web site contains a visiting nurse locator, caregiver information, and related links to other organizations.

### Hospice and Supportive Services

**Foundation for Hospice and Home Care**

National Association for Home Care
228 Seventh Street SE
Washington, DC 20003
Phone: 202-547-7424
Fax: 202-547-3540
Web site: *http://www.nahc.org*

This diverse organization offers a broad array of programs to serve the dying, disabled, and disadvantaged.

**Hospice Association of America (HAA)**

228 Seventh Street SE
Washington, DC 20003
Phone: 202-546-4759

Fax: 202-547-9559
Web site: *http://www.nahc.org/HAA/home.html*

This national trade association represents more than 2,800 hospices and thousands of caregivers and volunteers who serve terminally ill patients and their families. The HAA web site provides general information about hospice care, including a consumer's guide and a Bill of Rights for hospice patients.

**Hospice Education Institute/Hospicelink**
190 Westbrook Road
Essex, CT 06426
Toll-Free: 800-331-1620
Phone: 860-767-1620
Fax: 860-767-2746
E-mail: hospiceall@aol.com
Web site: *http://www.hospiceworld.org*

This not-for-profit organization provides general information and materials about hospice care and referrals to the hospice nearest you.

**Hospice Foundation of America (HFA)**
2001 S Street NW, Suite 300
Washington, DC 20009
Toll-Free: 800-854-3402
Fax: 202-638-5312
E-mail: hfa@hospicefoundation.org
Web site: *http://www.hospicefoundation.org*

The HFA offers information and materials on hospice care, a hospice locator service, and educational programs. The web site contains this information as well as links to related sites.

**Hospice Net**
Suite 51, 401 Bowling Avenue
Nashville, TN 37205
E-mail: comments@hospicenet.org
Web site: *http://www.hospicenet.org*

This nonprofit organization that works exclusively through the Internet provides articles regarding end-of-life issues. Hospice nurses, social workers, bereavement counselors, and chaplains are available to answer questions via e-mail. The web site includes information for patients and caregivers, information about grief and loss, and a hospice locator service.

**Joint Commission on Accreditation of Healthcare Organizations (JCAHO)**

One Renaissance Boulevard
Oakbrook Terrace, IL 60181
Toll-Free (questions regarding complaints only): 800-994-6610
Phone: 630-792-5000
Fax: 630-792-5005
Web site: *http://www.jcaho.org*

This nonprofit organization evaluates and accredits more than 19,500 health care organizations in the United States, including hospitals, health care networks and health care organizations that provide home care, long-term care, behavioral health care, laboratory, and ambulatory care services. JCAHO makes performance reports of accredited organizations and guidelines for choosing a health care facility available to the public.

**Medicare Helpline**

Department of Health and Human Services
Toll-Free: 800-MEDICAR (800-633-4227)
Web site: *http://www.medicare.gov*

Call the toll-free number to receive information about local Medicare services.

**National Association for Home Care (NAHC)**

228 Seventh Street SE
Washington, DC 20003
Phone: 202-547-7424
Fax: 202-547-3540
Web site: *http://www.nahc.org*

The NAHC provides a state-by-state database of phone numbers for home care and hospice agencies.

**National Hospice and Palliative Care Organization**

1700 Diagonal Road, Suite 300
Alexandria, VA 22314
Phone: 703-837-1500
E-mail: info@nhpco.org
Web site: *http://www.nhpco.org*

This organization is dedicated to providing information about hospice care. The web site contains related links, a hospice locator database by state, a newsletter, and other general information.

**Partnership for Caring, Inc.**

Program Office
475 Riverside Drive, Suite 1825
New York, NY 10115
Toll-Free: 800-989-WILL (800-989-9455)
Phone: 212-870-2003
Fax: 212-870-2040
E-mail: pfc@partnershipforcaring.org
Web site: *http://www.choices.org*

Partnership for Caring, Inc., formerly called Choice in Dying, is concerned with protecting the rights and serving the needs of people who are dying of any illness as well as the needs of their families. The organization distributes free information on living will and power of attorney and offers a free counseling service on end-of-life issues.

## Patient Education, Support, and Advocacy

*See also* the American Cancer Society Resources, pages 217–218.

**American Board of Medical Specialties**

1007 Church Street, Suite 404
Evanston, IL 60201-5913
Phone Verification: 866-ASK-ABMS (866-275-2267)
Phone: 847-491-9091
Fax: 847-328-3596
Web site: *http://www.abms.org*

The American Board of Medical Specialties (ABMS) is the umbrella organization for the twenty-four approved medical specialty boards in the United States. This organization provides information about specialization and certification in medicine. Their web site includes the Doctor Verification Service.

**American Self-Help Group Clearinghouse**

Northwest Covenant Medical Center
100 Hanover Avenue, Suite 202
Cedar Knolls, NJ 07927-2020
Phone: 973-326-6789
Fax: 973-306-9467
E-mail: njshc@bc.cybernex.net
Web site: *http://www.selfhelpgroups.org*

This group maintains a searchable database of over 1,000 self-help groups, including those concerning specific illnesses, caregivers, disabilities, and bereavement. It provides a referral service and helps people form their own groups.

**Burger King Cancer Caring Center**

4117 Liberty Avenue
Pittsburgh, PA 15224
Phone: 412-622-1212
Fax: 412-622-1216
E-mail: cancercr@sgi.net
Web site: *http://trfn.clpgh.org/cancercaring*

This center is dedicated to providing psychological support to people diagnosed with cancer and their families and friends. The Cancer Caring Center is now handling calls for the Cancer Guidance Hotline.

**Cancer Care, Inc.**

275 Seventh Avenue
New York, NY 10001
Toll-Free: 800-813-HOPE (800-813-4673)
Phone: 212-221-3300
Fax: 212-719-0263
E-mail: info@cancercare.org
Web site: *http://www.cancercare.org*

Cancer Care provides emotional and financial support for people with cancer and their families and educational programs for the general public. Free counseling, outreach programs, and information about and referrals for home care and child care, hospice, and other services are also available. *Spanish information is available on the web site.*

**Cancer Research Institute (CRI)**

681 Fifth Avenue
New York, NY 10022
Toll-Free: 800-99-CANCER (800-992-2623)
E-mail: info@cancerresearch.org
Web site: *http://www.cancerresearch.org*

An institute funding cancer research and providing public information on cancer immunology and cancer treatment, the CRI helps locate immunotherapy clinical trials, and offers a cancer reference guide and other informational booklets.

**Cancervive**

11636 Chayote Street
Los Angeles, CA 90049
Toll-Free: 800-4-TO-CURE (800-486-2873)
Phone: 310-203-9232
Fax: 310-471-4618
E-mail: cancervivr@aol.com
Web site: *http://www.cancervive.org*

Cancervive offers several services to people with cancer, including telephone counseling, referrals, and education.

***Coping with Cancer* Magazine**

PO Box 682268
Franklin, TN 37068-2268
Phone: 615-790-2400
Fax: 615-794-0179
E-mail: copingmag@aol.com
Web site: *http://www.copingmag.com*

This bimonthly publication is the only nationally distributed consumer magazine for people whose lives have been touched by cancer.

**Make Today Count**

Care of Neil O'Connor
K4-B100, CSC
UW Hospital and Clinics
600 Highland Avenue
Madison, WI 53792
Phone: 608-263-8521
E-mail: njoconnor@hosp.wisc.edu
Web site: *http://userpages.itis.com/lemoll/index.html*

This support organization is for people affected by cancer or other life-threatening illness.

**The Mautner Project for Lesbians with Cancer**

1707 L Street NW, Suite 500
Washington, DC 20036
Phone (TTY): 202-332-5536
Fax: 202-332-0662
E-mail: mautner@mautnerproject.org
Web site: *http://www.mautnerproject.org*

This group provides vital services and support, including education, information, and advocacy for health issues relating to lesbians with cancer and their families.

**The National Coalition for Cancer Research (NCCR)**

426 C Street NE
Washington, DC 20002
Phone: 202-544-1880 (ask for NCCR)
Web site: *http://www.cancercoalition.org*

Through NCCR, cancer survivors and researchers track cancer research and monitor legislation and funding.

**National Coalition for Cancer Survivorship (NCCS)**

1010 Wayne Avenue, Suite 770
Silver Spring, MD 20910-5600
Toll-Free: 877-NCCS-YES (877-622-7937)
Phone: 301-650-9127
Fax: 301-565-9670
Web site: *http://www.cansearch.org*
Web site (Spanish version): *http://www.cansearch.org/spanish/index.html*

The NCCS is a network of independent organizations working in the area of cancer survivorship and support. The web site offers links to on-line cancer resources, support groups, survivorship programs, advocacy education, and a newsletter.

**National Self-Help Clearinghouse**

Graduate School and University Center of the City University of New York
365 Fifth Avenue, Suite 3300
New York, NY 10016
Phone: 212-817-1822
Fax: 212-817-2990
Web site: *http://www.selfhelpweb.org*

This nonprofit organization provides access to regional self-help services.

**National Women's Health Network**

514 Tenth Street NW, Suite 400
Washington, DC 20004
Phone: 202-628-7814
Fax: 202-347-1168
Web site: *http://www.womenshealthnetwork.org*

This organization provides advocacy and maintains a clearinghouse on women's health issues.

**Oncolink's Coping with Cancer**

Web site: *http://www.oncolink.upenn.edu/psychosocial*

Maintained by the University of Pennsylvania Cancer Center, this web site includes information about several different kinds of support groups and other issues that many people with cancer may encounter.

**People Living Through Cancer**

323 Eighth Street SW
Albuquerque, NM 87102
Toll-Free: 888-441-4439
Phone: 505-242-3263
Fax: 505-242-6756
Web site: *http://www.pltc.org*

Programs and activities to help members make informed choices and interact with other people who have been treated for cancer. Services include a publication, one-to-one matching, support groups and individual counseling, and training for Native Americans who would like to start their own groups.

**Pharmaceutical Research and Manufacturers Association of America (PhRMA)**

1100 Fifteenth Street NW, Suite 900
Washington, DC 20005
Phone: 202-835-3400
Fax: 202-835-3414
Web site: *http://www.phrma.org*

The PhRMA provides information about member pharmaceutical companies and drugs that are currently available, in clinical trials, or under development. The web site includes a directory of patient assistance programs for prescription drugs and a database of new medications for cancer and other diseases.

**Social Security Administration**

Office of Public Inquiries
6401 Security Boulevard, Room 4-C-5 Annex
Baltimore, MD 21235-6401
Toll-Free: 800-772-1213
Toll-Free (TTY): 800-325-0778
Web site: *http://www.ssa.gov*

Call the toll-free number to receive information about local services. *Spanish-speaking staff is available.*

**The Wellness Community**

35 E. Seventh Street, Suite 412
Cincinnati, OH 45202-2420
Toll-Free: 888-793-WELL (888-793-9355)
Phone: 513-421-7111
Fax: 513-421-7119
Web site: *http://www.wellness-community.org*

This free program offers support for people with cancer and their loved ones. The nonprofit organization provides professional support services as an adjunct to conventional medical treatment in twenty-six facilities nationwide. Services include support groups, networking groups for specific types of cancer, educational workshops, stress management sessions, lectures, and social gatherings. Support groups are led by licensed psychotherapists.

# INDEX

Page numbers in **boldface** refer to highlights of specific cancers. Page numbers in *italic* refer to illustrations.

# About the Author

Edward H. Laughlin, MD, FACS is Professor of Surgery, University of Alabama at Birmingham, Huntsville Program. He was the first chairman of the surgical program, and has been engaged in teaching for over a quarter century. A graduate of Duke University School of Medicine, he interned at the Johns Hopkins Hospital and completed his residency in general surgery at the University of Virginia Hospital. He is the author of numerous papers in peer-reviewed journals, and memberships include the Society of Surgical Oncology and the American Society of Clinical Oncology.